UNLOCKED

DISCOVERING YOUR HIDDEN KEYS

CARMELLE CRINNION

DAWN PUBLISHING

© 2020 Carmelle Crinnion

Published by Dawn Publishing
www.dawnbates.com
The moral right of the author has been asserted.

For quantity sales or media enquiries, please contact the publisher at the website address above.

Cataloguing-in-Publication entry is available from the British Library.

ISBN:
978-1-913973-05-6 (paperback)
978-1-913973-06-3 (ebook)
978-1-913973-09-4 (audiobook)

Book cover design – Miladinka Milic

All rights reserved. No part of this book may be reproduced, stored in a retrieval system, communicated or transmitted in any form or by means without written permission. All inquiries should be made to the publisher at the above address.

Disclaimer: The material in this publication is of the nature of general comment only and does not represent professional advice. It is not intended to provide specific guidance for particular circumstances and should not be relied on as the basis for any decision to take action or not to take action on any matters which it covers.

ALSO PUBLISHED BY DAWN PUBLISHING

Becoming Annie – The Biography of a Curious Woman

by Dawn Bates (2020)

Moana – One Woman's Journey Back to Self

by Dawn Bates (2020)

Becoming the Champion – V1 Awareness

by Korey Carpenter (2020)

The Trilogy of Life Itself:

Friday Bridge – Becoming a Muslim, Becoming Everyone's Business

by Dawn Bates (2nd Edition, 2017)

Walaahi – A firsthand account of living through the Egyptian Uprising and why I walked away from Islaam

by Dawn Bates (2017)

Crossing The Line – A Journey of Purpose and Self-Belief

by Dawn Bates (2017)

This book is dedicated to you, the reader.
May you unlock your truth and realise your potential is unlimited.

CONTENTS

Foreword — ix
Gratitude — xiii

1. The Beginning — 1
2. Conversations and Confidence — 7
3. My First Love — 13
4. Sydney Life, Babies and Marriage — 25
5. The Years with My Girls — 31
6. Andrew, Marriage and Business — 35
7. The Business Journey — 41
8. Triathlon — 45
9. Strength Training and Body Shaping — 53
10. Sameha And Marianne — 59
11. The Next Upgrade — 75
12. Separation — 79
13. The Innocence of Spirit In Children — 87
14. Harsh Lessons and Disruption — 95
15. Machu Picchu 2012 — 101
16. The Floodgates Open — 111
17. Egypt 2015 — 117
18. The Nile Cruise — 121
19. Kundalini Rising — 127
20. Dances of Inception — 133
21. Working with Clients — 137
22. Trust, Forgiveness and Jealousy — 143
23. Sexual Healing – A Journey — 155
24. Dating in the Modern World — 165
25. Breast Implants – Worst Decision Ever — 171
26. Ding Ding – Wait – What? — 181

Unlocked — 187
About the Author — 191
Dawn Publishing — 193

FOREWORD

Understanding who we are as individuals, couples and communities, as well as our relationship to one another, is something that has baffled philosophers and psychologists for a long time.

Attend any university around the world and you will find multiple courses on the subjects of humanity, the mind, the 'mind, body, spirit' connection, not to mention relationships, the human body and you have to dive into religion, spirituality and theology sections of the book stores or libraries to even get close to what it may mean to be human, spiritual or enlightened.

To understand our bodies we have come to rely on men in white coats, and in the last decade or two women in white coats, but do any of them actually truly understand the full capacity, preferring to focus more on the academic, the blinkered view of what they feel they must write to have their thesis awarded a pass, or to avoid being seen as a 'quack' who faces being ostracised from the medical field.

It is only when we read the real life stories of those who have truly understood the connection with each part of themselves, done the research, explored their mind, body and soul, and allowed themselves to be open to what is truly possible that any of us begin to feel any amount of permission to question what the scholars and the medics tell us.

Only when we read the true stories of those who are brave enough to make a stand, to share in all their vulnerability, expose their own mistakes and misunderstandings that any of us can have the permission and the confidence to speak our own truths against these so called experts in the world.

No one knows us more than we know ourselves, and yet we hand over permission time and time again to people who really have no idea about what it is we are experiencing, then choosing to follow scripted flowcharts or revelations based on culture or tradition.

Only when we question the authorities, only when we question ourselves, with the really deep confronting questions can we actually begin to understand our place in the world, what we stand for, and then start to unravel the beauty of life itself.

By healing our wounds of the past, in this life or another, or the ones passed down to us from generation to generation, we get to see ourselves from a more enriching perspective – and not just enriching for us, but our children, our parents, siblings, neighbours and humanity as a whole.

By choosing to see, and be confronted by, the damage we are doing to others, to ourselves, we learn more and more about the problems facing society today, and this is why Carmelle's journey into discovering who and why she is who she is, and why her gifts are so important in the healing of this world is a story that needs to be shared.

For us to truly understand the damaging impact that unquestioning belief in the doctors and medical world as a whole has on us all, because they are no better equipped to learn and decipher information than we are, we need to do our research, we need to question everything we are told by them, and by the religious institutions of the world.

We need to question everything, because when we have faith in ourselves, in our Creator, whatever kind of entity we believe that to be, then the Divine faith gifted to us from the moment our souls were created, will deliver us all the answers we are truly looking for, not within the walls of academia, but in the sharing of our journeys, our experiences and our learnings.

Carmelle's story is one which runs deep in every human being on the planet on some level, and it isn't unique to culture, ethnicity, nationality, or faith. It is human; and the more we ignore the truth of who we are, and why we are the way we are, the more we damage ourselves and humans as a whole.

This is a brave story, and the bravery resides within all of us, if only we will allow it to.

I am deeply honoured to have been part of Carmelle's journey, a journey of immense personal growth, courage and resilience. For her to gift you this book has taken her to the depths of her soul, made her face fears she didn't even know she had, and awaken other parts of herself she was not aware of; and she did it so she could serve humanity – not from ego, but from love. Love of self, love of being of service, and a love of love itself.

It has been a rollercoaster ride of epic proportions and she has ridden it well, incredibly well.

Carmelle, I am so very proud of you my darling, and I just know this is the start of a new and very beautiful journey into being of service to others on a whole new level; one I know you are more than ready for.

With love for you, and to you, my Doyenne,

Your coach, friend and soul sister,

Dawn

Dawn Bates
International Bestselling Author, Author Coach and Strategist, Publisher, Molecule Shaking Speaker and Activist.
www.dawnbates.com

GRATITUDE

This book would not have been possible without the guidance of my author coach and life coach, Dawn Bates. This woman took a dream that I had and – through countless sessions – she drilled into my psyche to reveal the content I knew I had to share and helped me to unravel some sticking points along the way. So, Dawn, from the bottom of my heart, thank you.

My children Angela, Emily, Ryan and Daniel have all been very supportive albeit inquisitive about the content of my book, and to them, I wouldn't have much of the content of this book if it wasn't for you guys. So I love you and I thank you for your unconditional love and support.

My mum has been a constant inspiration throughout my life and continues to be to this day at the age of 88. Mum has never judged or criticised any choice I've made, has always offered me priceless advice and I would be lost without her to talk to. Thanks for always being there for me Mum, I love you.

To my siblings and in-laws John, Karen, Tim, Paola, Michelle and Andrew, thanks for always lighting up my life on our somewhat irregular get-togethers with laughter and memories and a little wine. It's all helped in the writing of this book.

My close friends Julie, Jen, Dan, Hulya, you've listened to me and encouraged me to follow my dream of getting this book published. Thanks for being there for me.

To the publishing and creative team of Dawn Publishing, you're awesome! Thank you.

ONE
THE BEGINNING

What I'm about to tell you is the story of how my life changed radically, in the space of just a moment in time, in the lull in between my thoughts, in that little space of nothingness where magic finds its way without resistance. From that moment on I would never be the same, and my life would become a playground for my spiritual journey where I would explore worlds I thought I never knew existed. Of course, I did know they existed; I had just forgotten – like we all have. I was entering the place where I would access ancient memories and bring them forth to create from a place of unlimited potential, and it would be my job to share this with the world if I chose to do so.

On one ordinary day in January 2012 I was driving my car to work, not necessarily thinking about anything in particular, when something peculiar happened. I began speaking, but the words I spoke were not coming from my own conscious thoughts and I hadn't planned on talking out loud to myself. I just simply began speaking, and this is how it went.

M: We are ready to speak through you now.
C: Who is this?
M: It is I, Mother.
C: Okay.

I stumbled, not knowing what to say but desperately wanting to keep the conversation going. The sensation was bizarre as I began speaking from both participants of the conversation.

M: We are ready to teach you our language. You are to use it in your healing sessions. You are ready.
C: So, you're going to speak through me?
M: Yes.
C: You're going to teach me a language?
M: Yes.

And that was the extent of my first conversation. I was beaming and just so happy. My fascination with spirituality had begun in the previous couple of years and I had been listening to the conversations of the spiritual channel Abraham Hicks for many months. I was in awe of the clear channel that Esther Hicks was for the spiritual collective known as Abraham. Their messages were life changing for me in that I was discovering a whole way of living and being than the one I had been used to. Many aspects of my life had opened up for review since I began tapping into this fascinating world. It seemed to me to hold answers that I had been searching my whole life for. And now, here I was doing exactly what had held such alluring enchantment and delight for me. I was beyond excited, and also a little apprehensive at the sheer magnitude I knew was unfolding.

My car seemed to be the classroom for these spiritual downloads and lessons. I slowly began to work out how to allow the consciousness of spirit speak through me. If I focused on what was actually happening too much I would stumble and feel like I was gagging. When I was resistant because of being in my head too much at the sheer weirdness of what was happening, it was as if my whole mouth would fill up with words only for me to finally blurt them out in a stilted language, like I was verbally vomiting. I began getting used to the vibrational rise in my chest, traveling up and through my trachea like a wave rising into my throat and out of my mouth.

It's important to also know that I had been communicating before this time with Mother, which is why I was familiar, relieved and awestruck at our conversation. Our communication had been through involuntary movements of my body, so I had learned long before this to allow my body to receive communication from her, nonverbal communication, more energetic so that I would feel myself actually embodying the essence of this aspect that I now was. It began in the early days of my spiritual awareness, only around two years prior, which I will go into in detail a little further into the book.

The tricky part was forming words in a foreign language that is not spoken by others. Learning to roll my 'r's at certain times while trying not to sound like a robot in the delivery of the words, proved to be a huge challenge. I soon learned to relax my body and allow my mind to be open so that in the nanosecond from non-spoken to spoken word, I became skilled enough to pronounce beautifully sounding words, then sentences and whole dialogues.

I often broke off mid-sentence to go over and over certain words and pronunciations until I projected them 'just so'. I was not going to get away with being lazy in the elocution department, and I sensed there was to be a certain tone, as well as presence when this was to be delivered. The pitch was also important, as was the tempo. At certain times, the pitch was very high, sometimes very low, and I could feel the shift in the vibrational frequency when the pitch was adjusted. At first the speaking was at what I would consider to be a normal speaking pace, but later I found that this was a part of the learning process, as with any learning process it was going through stages and creating a foundational vocabulary from which to expand exponentially only months later.

I wasn't meant to be able to interpret this dialogue directly into English, that's not what this was about, and I learned this quickly enough. The language is so powerful and carries such a high vibration that it doesn't need any translation to feel the effect upon you when you hear it. I went on to learn that we were originally vibrational beings who needed no words to convey our thoughts to one another, the vibration was enough. Now I was learning the importance in feeling into the actual energy around the dialogue, taking in the essence without focusing on it making sense in the moment.

As time went by and I became at one with this language, I was more easily able to allow my entire being to bring through the actual sensation, the presence of the flow of dialogue. My facial expressions would change dramatically as I spoke, sometimes conveying pain, sadness or extreme happiness and laughing. My whole-body language spoke loudly of the emotions and sentiment in the colloquy, almost like I was delivering a message to the person in front of me, and it was imperative that I convey the tone perfectly.

I would learn that the language of Light is an information conduit. The words and sounds are formed via a high vibrational connection to the surrounding codes which are constantly around us, and constantly moving, upgrading, swirling, shape shifting – working with the Divine source which is the creator of this Universe. Since we came here in the knowing we would forget everything, with the intention of remembering and then challenging ourselves to become more highly creative, this was a gift we could use to connect with the higher consciousness that we so easily drift away from when 'life' happens.

An incredible addition to my gifts was that my voice was transformed into a most magnificent singing voice. And since I had never been able to hold even the most basic of tunes this was quite a pleasant yet bewildering surprise to me, and then to my family, friends and clients – once I was confident enough to allow them to hear.

Later, I had a client who was a music teacher, her passion for music was her life. She was in her sixties, raising her granddaughter as her own child due to family circumstances. We had many sessions together and during this time I was only just bringing through my voice. As the months went by, I was becoming more connected and synthesised to this extension of my vocal range. As we were chatting after our session one day, she said she had been in awe of how I reached all of the octaves of all the notes. I'm pretty sure she thought I was hiding a secret musical degree I had, or a secret life as a musician! She had a keenly developed auditory perception and was genuinely praising and honouring my skill, even though she was aware that I was bringing through a divinely prepared score, uniquely for her healing and transformation.

Upon reflection, of course she was going to receive a perfectly orchestrated vocal range, since that's what tone she carried in her own vibration. Her healings with me were an extension of her deeply integrated knowing that her tone was in need of a fine tune from the

Divine, while also honouring her passion and appreciation for musical perfection.

By this stage I had been given countless 'singing lessons'. Most of these were when I was driving, I would continually practise bringing different tones through, learning how to hold my tongue, how to purse or soften my lips, how to manipulate the back of my throat, how to breathe to prepare for long, often very long notes.

The ancient languages I channel – there are many dialects – have a history that predates our Earth. But in fact, they exist on all dimensions, meaning they are in the past, the present and the future. The language of the Spirit. The way the words, phrases and tones are formed, and then woven into my own voice through unconditional trust and allowing, creates the perfect framework for Universal codes to form. It's something like a spiders web with golden orbs filled with information, ready for expansion at the perfect moments. The tones can release the messages within the golden orbs. There is no limit to what can be healed.

My eyes also play a very large part in the healing sessions. I see this spiders web energy field around the body of my client in a one on one setting, and then my eyes take over the next intricate segment of the process. At this stage my eyes move at lightning speed, darting from point to point in this domain of energy, connecting, disconnecting, weaving and threading energetic discords, imbalances and disharmonies, along with unhooking and disassembling the knots that bind old and outdated beliefs and stories from their very foundation. It would be literally impossible for me to try to move my eyes in this manner voluntarily. In fact, I have experienced many, many moments of eye work where my eyes actually circle around in opposing directions. The power of the eye muscles is incredible, and I have only found this through allowing this extension of myself through the union of a higher consciousness.

I was ready for my true soul purpose to reign supreme in my life! I was reassured by my trusted spiritual constant, Mother, that the flood gates were about to open, that people would seek me out, find me and I would work this magic with them.

Even though it was Mother who I identified with, I recognise the importance of searching for this understanding and perspective for me to continue doing this work. If I couldn't have a conversation on the level I was used to, as a human – knowing who I was speaking with, being able to ask questions and receive answers in the language I knew – then it would have been difficult or even impossible for me to proceed. It would become difficult to continue at the level of trust that was required, had I not had this touch and warmth through familiar words, albeit between spirit and human/spirit. As time has progressed and my everyday life includes this practice, I feel so comfortable with the languages I channel and the knowledge I have, I often forget other people aren't living with this gift, and that's the truest way I can describe it. I've had a private tutor, internally in my subconscious, and over the past eight years I have nurtured the lessons, the language and the way of life so that it's now integrated into my being.

Like anything new, you become accustomed to it and forget how it came to being, the desire which manifested it, and then the devotion to the craft of choice that filled you with excitement and anticipation to learn more and more.

And this desire then fuels more questions, which in turn create more answers at the next level you're now ready for.

It's the thirst for knowledge, for anything and everything, that brings us the raw material to firstly acknowledge and then to integrate a part of ourselves into.

TWO
CONVERSATIONS AND CONFIDENCE

My quest and desire has not waned since the very first moment I felt the connection to this highest aspect of me. In fact, I remember many years ago when I was probably around 10 years old, feeling what was probably the seed being planted for this life I am now living.

I was in Mass one morning – I was raised in the Catholic religion – and after Holy Communion, recited a prayer which I had come to know and feel was my receiving of the blessings of Jesus and the Holy Spirit in my soul.

In this moment, and many subsequent times like this, I felt such a calmness, such a belonging, such a place of peace and love that it felt like home, like Heaven on Earth. I loved to visit this place, and reciting this prayer took me there.

> *Soul of Christ*
> *Be my sanctification*
> *Body of Christ*
> *Be my salvation*
> *Blood of Christ*
> *Fill my veins*
> *Water of Christ's side*

Wash out my stains
Passion of Christ
My comfort be
Oh, good Jesus,
Listen to me
In thy wounds I fain would hide
Ne'er to be parted from thy side
Guard me should the foe assail me
Call me when my life shall fail me
Bid me come to thee above
With thy saints to sing thy love
World without end
Amen.

I loved being in that place so much that I began accompanying my mum to early morning masses during the week. I was the only one of the four of us kids who was crazy enough to want to get out of bed before I actually had to on a school morning. It was on one such morning that I met who I consider to be my first spiritual teacher. A sister of St Joseph, one of the many who lived in the accompanying convent next to the church and school of St Columbkilles in Corrimal, New South Wales.

She approached my mum and myself after Mass one morning and asked if I would like to do some of the readings since it was always the same people on the pulpit every morning. It would be nice to see a fresh young face. Well, I loved the idea, but my reading skills and confidence needed a little honing, so she began coaching me. The simplistic tips she gave me resulted in confidence to stand in front of the congregation, small as it was, and read beautifully. Pause for one second at every comma, for two seconds at each full stop. Don't rush. This is something I have carried with me all my life, emphasise the pauses not only in reading but in life, slow it down. It's such a beautiful thing and it made the experience very pleasurable. I loved those mornings. I can't remember how long we continued attending but it left an indelible imprint on my heart.

Why was I ready to begin such a life changing journey?

In the year prior to the conversation in the car with Mother, my constant mantra was, "I release all that no longer serves me". I believe this allowed me to heal myself of much of my emotional trauma, the old stories and baggage that kept me from connecting to my soul. I had spent too long feeling soulless. In fact, I had been so extremely distraught at my own disconnection, feeling like I didn't know what was best for me in even the smallest of decisions, that in desperation one day I declared out loud, in private, "I don't have a soul" and furthermore that I would be better off leaving decisions to others to make for me, since they seemed to know what was best for me.

Saying those words felt like speaking the truth, and – to be perfectly transparent – I felt relieved. Relieved of the burden of anguish and disconnection to myself. This was the first step towards taking ownership of the direction of my life, and even though it felt like I was taking the easy way out, I was opening a Pandora's box of healing and unexplored potential.

From a psychological point of view there were some straightforward methods of approaching and moving through this. I would find out soon enough via counseling and therapy that I had been in the habit of people pleasing for many, many years by this time. Of course, I knew how I felt but I had never gone deep enough with inner inquiry to find out what my patterns were to enable me to address them. I went from relationship to relationship without taking any time to reflect on where things had gone wrong, beyond the symptoms and reasons that were literally only the clues to the deeper work I needed to do. It's all too easy to fall back into old patterns of behaviour even after initially showing signs of change.

It wasn't at all intentional that I didn't take the time to be alone, and not in a relationship, I felt it was very synchronistic that as I came out of one relationship, I met the next amazing man who would seem perfect for me. I didn't think or know that there was a whole lot that I needed to address deep down in order to enter into a healthy balanced relationship. When you go from an unhappy relationship into forming a new one, there is so much encouragement from everyone around you, its simply what society thinks is a wonderful progression. The reality is that the load you carry from previous relationships still sits heavily on your shoulders, in your heart and in your soul, unhealed and silently accumulating more evidence to cling tightly to old patterns when they eventually rise again, because they do.

I had been offering myself on a platter to my current partner and the ones before him for as long as I could remember, often figuratively saying – help yourself – in every way: mentally, physically, emotionally. I often felt overridden in conversations, I had allowed myself to believe that he/they knew so much more than me and I would be a better person for listening and learning from them.

I did learn much from my relationships. I grew and became confident in many ways, experiencing world travel, a great social life, financial stability (notwithstanding how it was tested in my last marriage) and freedom, as well as becoming a mother, an athlete and a businesswoman. It's truly amazing how functional, normal and wonderful one's life can be while there are deeper and destructive underlying programs running areas of your life, just lying dormant until triggered.

My behaviour was a result of much deeper childhood issues in my subconscious, running the inner dialogue which went something like, *Carmelle, don't take up too much space or attention, stay small because something bad might happen if you are too needy or cause trouble.*

In doing this I would allow the most important people in my life to lead the way in many important decisions, taking their opinions as being the right choice for me. I would cower away from conflict, my mind would go blank, I would become extremely emotional, I would feel the rise of fear in my stomach if confronted or even if I was asked to prove myself regarding an opinion. It was so much easier to let the other person be right if I was tested.

Often, I felt threatened by others in relation to failing to live up to their expectations, which was all in my own head, yet those inner conversations were very loud and very real. I was a very convincing voice in my subconscious. In reality I was not living up to my own expectations, but I didn't know how to do that, so I kept the inner dialogue which kept me stuck in a place of complacency and submission, yet longing and desire to be better.

The irony of all of this is that I wanted to be seen! I wanted people to listen to me, I wanted to be known. I'm a Taurus woman and I have a deep desire to walk this earth with my head held high, speaking from a place of confidence and authority. For years there was a battle going on between the hushed version of myself and the version that loved attention and being seen. It was torture inside. I surrounded myself with people who were brilliant, who were extroverts, and who had confidence and who also had a circle of friends who were similar. For years I learned from all of these people and my inner confidence grew to a large extent. I loved being around such incredible high achievers and lovers of life, they lifted me up.

So with this little piece of insight I will now take you through the journey and the accompanying stories of my significant relationships, and how I desperately wanted to just be happy and content with what I had, whilst living and growing as my family grew.

THREE
MY FIRST LOVE

I decided to leave school at the end of Year 11 to go to business college. I could see no sense in completing my Higher School Certificate since I definitely didn't want to study for another four years. I just wanted to work, earn some money and have the freedom that I would find with having my own money.

As well as college, I had two casual jobs, one at a jewellery store which was pretty boring, and the other was at a squash centre, owned by one of my best friend's parents.

I quickly picked up a racquet and began playing squash and put myself down to play in the weekly teams' competitions. It soon became a place I spent a lot of time practising, playing and working. One of my shifts was Sunday from nine to five, and after arriving one Sunday and settling in, a guy entered the front door. He had a really high energy around him, so happy, friendly and fun.

Before I knew what was happening, he was around my side of the counter crouching down, apparently searching for his racquet and began play-biting my leg! I didn't know what was happening and was jumping around carrying on and laughing telling him to stop. He was pretty charming and just so electric. That was the first time I met Greg.

He asked me to go out to dinner with him the following week, and I said yes. He was 25 and I was only 17 and fresh out of school, it felt good being around him. He could easily carry conversation and had lots of stories to tell and I definitely felt an attraction to him. He thought I was wonderful and encouraged me to be more adventurous and inquisitive in life.

Greg quickly became my knight in shining armour. He showed me the world that existed outside of my own limited scope, a world of fun and adventure. We travelled, we spent weekends outdoors doing all kinds of different sports and hanging out with others who loved the same lifestyle. We would sail on his catamaran, go water skiing and stay at our friends cabin down the coast, go snow skiing in the winter as many weekends as we could, play squash regularly, literally squeezing as much fun into our lives as possible. I fell in love with this life.

He proposed on my 19th birthday and we were married less than a year later, just before I turned 20.

By this time, we had purchased a home together which we moved straight into once we were married, it was in a beautiful location only a short stroll to the beach. Early married life saw me settle right into becoming a home maker, cooking, baking and making our house feel very welcoming and warm. It was as I'd imagined, or rather it was exactly how I expected life to unfold. Get married, have children and live happily ever after.

My glory box had been gradually filled with sheets, towels, kitchen items and appliances, all manner of trinkets, all purchased in the few years prior with the very handy lay-bye system. In fact, at least half of my income was spent on paying off these lay byes. It was what we were taught to do to prepare for when we did marry and move out of home. My sister Michelle and I loved coming home with new items to show each other and Mum, adding them to the growing booty we each had. Michelle was engaged too and was to be married just a few months before me.

Then something very unexpected transpired when only six months into our marriage we relocated to Papua New Guinea. Greg was brilliant in his field not only as an accountant but in the emerging computer age. He had an inquisitive genius mind and very quickly became a wiz at programming, thus becoming highly sought after, as it turned out not only in our own hometown but offshore as well.

We discussed it seriously and came to the conclusion that he would go to PNG first and see what it was like living there for a month or so, and also if he was happy with the job. If everything was going well and he was happy, I would resign from my full-time job and join him. We had already packed up and rented out our home and I was staying with Mum and Dad. We talked often over those weeks and made the decision to make PNG our home for a couple of years. So I resigned, packed my bags and boarded my flight to start a new and very exciting chapter of my life.

When I first arrived in Mount Hagen, flying into Kagamuga airport, a tiny strip outside the main town, I was greeted by Greg who was absolutely thrilled to see me. He took me straight to our new home which was literally across the road from the airport in a small block of six apartments. There was no looking back, we loved it from the first day. We made friends with our Kiwi neighbours pretty quickly and began exploring the social life that the expats from all over the world enjoyed while working here.

My first job started only three days after arriving, a temporary position for six weeks doing clerical work at a coffee company. The highlands of PNG are filled with tea and coffee plantations so there were plenty of expats working in this industry. In fact, we lived on a plantation for at least one year during our stay and it was a wonderful lifestyle. The plantation had about five homes dotted around the property, and a pool, tennis court and entertainment area for us all to enjoy.

Our circle of friends grew, and we played squash in a small complex a few times a week. We joined a running group called Hash House Harriers which is an international group of non-competitive runners who organise HHH events.

Our group had a weekly run which went something like this. The hosts of the week would go out ahead of the run and map it out. At random points on the run they would place circles of white flour on the ground which would indicate there is a choice of direction to take, and it might go in two or three different directions. They would place a further two flour circles on the correct path only. So, when the runners got to these points they would split up and when the correct path was established by finding the next two flour circles, that runner would call out HASH HASH loudly to let the others know.

It was a lot of fun, and being the highlands of a third world country, there were plenty of bush tracks with creeks, grass huts and small villages along the way.

At the end of the run, the hosts would invite us to their house for a sausage sizzle and beer. Since this was the 80s – before all the technology we have today – our social life was crucial, and we depended on each other to create the most fun and adventurous times we could. Two couples we spent a lot of time with were from New Zealand and we had the most epic dinner parties.

Most expats had cooks and house cleaners supplied by their employers, so we had lots of free time to socialise. Our weekends were times to chill or explore or both. Many Sundays were spent by the pool at our friend's place in Banz, a small town about 30 minutes' drive away. This was most always after an indulgent Saturday night eating the feast prepared by their cook, sitting by the open fire since the nights were always cool, and drinking imported German beer and apple Schnapps, a favourite in our little circle of friends.

I have always enjoyed cooking so opted to not have a cook boi or meri (boy or girl), and instead to experiment with my own skills. Before long I was asking Mum and my sister Michelle to send over more Women's Weekly cookbooks which were my favourites. I loved the Italian one the most, and we ate like royalty with three course meals being the norm when we entertained. I would never even have thought of having people over without serving them three courses.

In one of my letters to Mum and Dad, to whom I wrote weekly, I told them of a dinner party the previous night where I served asparagus crepes with béchamel sauce, then apricot stuffed lamb with potato bake and veggies, followed by fried ice cream and banana fritters. It sounds like a feast from Viking times and I wonder now how we stuffed ourselves with so much food, and rich food at that. I only cooked like this for dinner parties though, the rest of the time we ate very health consciously and much lighter.

On two occasions we went to a place called Kiap Lodge. It was an eco-lodge in an isolated location in the jungle and we needed to take a very sturdy four-wheel drive for the journey through thick and rough terrain to get there. But boy it was worth it. It was so tranquil, so beautiful. It was named after the orchids that grew there, so was often referred to as Orchid Lodge. Homemade everything resulted in the most organic and delicious food I had ever tasted. I took the recipe for the bread they made and continued making that bread for the duration of our stay there in PNG.

Another time we climbed PNG's tallest mountain, Mt Wilhelm – a 4509 metre summit. We drove to the base camp and walked at a pretty leisurely pace before setting up camp for the night.

There was quite a group, maybe a dozen of us from memory, and we all contributed to making dinner that night. It turned into a big pot stew consisting of everything including beans – a big mistake. Needless to say, none of us wanted to be downwind from the group when we set off in the morning. Farting aside, we got up very early to climb for the next few hours, reaching the summit at sunrise.

It was spectacular, the views were stunning as the sun rose quickly, turning everything into a magical wonderland. It was extremely windy and cold at the top and there was a visitors' book attached to a rock so that we could enter our names and country of origin. As we opened the book, pages flew out everywhere!!! Oh no! We didn't bother putting our names in, or maybe we did, I can't remember, but we had such a great time with our expat friends, as we did on so many occasions.

During our second year living abroad we took six weeks leave and travelled to Europe for a five-week skiing holiday, meeting up with my dear friend from primary school days Debbie and her husband in Switzerland for a few days travelling in their campervan.

I recall one night we were driving in the van after spending the day in Austria exploring the most beautiful sights and taking in so much incredible history, we even went inside the famous glass house from *The Sound of Music* where Leisl sings 'I am 16 going on 17'. It was getting late and dark. We had no plans on where to stay the night, so we decided to pull over and spend the night in what seemed a peaceful location just off the road.

When we woke up the next morning, we found we were perched on the side of the most magnificent mountain with views that took our breath away. I'll never forget that morning, it was like waking up inside a dream.

After parting ways, we continued our skiing holiday with a little time for some significant historical sites, before returning home to Mount Hagen.

In between jobs I wanted to be occupied in my spare time, so I put out word that I was quite handy with a sewing machine, which I had brought with me – it was a birthday present from my mother-in-law. Word got around in the bush telegraph and I was soon asked to make curtains for a large home on a homestead for a wealthy Australian property owner who permanently resided there. I hadn't sewn curtains before, so I took on the job and just learned as I went. It was a large job, but I enjoyed doing it and seeing the finished product, and I earned some money as well.

Even when I was working, I spent many hours making my own clothes. Mum and my sister Michelle had the job of finding more patterns and material to send to me so I could keep adding to my wardrobe which was minimal. I was in need of cool dresses, skirts and tops to wear to work and when we went out.

When I read the letters I'd sent home, which thankfully Mum has kept all these years, I'm reminded of just how full our lives were. We both worked full time including half days on Saturday, played squash at least twice a week, I did 90 minutes of aerobics every day after work, we ran once or twice a week, swam laps in the plantation pool, I sewed not only for other people, but also made our own curtains and bedspread and pillow slips and also a hand sewn patchwork quilt. We maintained the grounds around the pool since the plantation owners didn't do a very good job at that time and we used the area regularly.

The second job that fell into my lap was at Mount Hagen technical college, as a teacher for typing and bookkeeping. The job had become available when the previous teacher left without notice so there was an urgency to find a replacement. Someone I knew asked me if I would apply for it, but since I had only ever done a three-month basic typing course at business college, I knew I was under qualified. And not only in my abilities – I was a great typist but knew nothing about bookkeeping – I was not a qualified teacher.

Somehow, I landed the job since it was convenient to have the position filled without having to go through the hiring process and then waiting to have that person move to a new country to take up the position. The salary was great, and the work was so much fun! I literally learned the lessons I was going to teach on the evening prior to teaching them.

I learned that these students were after a basic education, teaching them fundamental skills while respecting their village life. During class it was common to have students batting at their head, then pulling out nits and squashing them – so funny.

They taught me as much as I taught them, and some of the girls made me a billum, a string bag they wove which is used extensively all over the country to carry loads of food to and from the markets, as well as to carry babies. It is tied and hung from the forehead and hangs down to their lower back. I wanted to bring that memento home with me, made with bare hands in a remote village and infused with such love. I also collected several of the beautiful woven baskets they are famous for.

My diet changed significantly while living in the highlands. I eliminated meat several months after arriving, after seeing the trays of meat in the supermarket black around the edges. The availability of fresh produce made it easy to become more plant based, and then I read a book by Nathan Pritikin and was quickly converted to adhering strictly to the Pritikin diet. It was very strict and almost no fat was included. I actually loved eating that way, and before long – not that I needed to lose weight – I was at the leanest I've ever been and feeling absolutely fantastic and very fit.

Not only had I been running and playing squash, but I had brought a video of the Jane Fonda workout with me. There weren't many days I missed doing these aerobic and flexibility workouts and was soon up to easily doing the 90-minute challenge workout daily, after work.

One day I received a letter from Mum saying that a second cousin on Dad's side who lived in England, had a son who was coming from England to work – of all places – in Mount Hagen. So, both the distant cousin, however many times removed, and I were both given each other's details, and eventually met up when he arrived with his wife. Paul and Allison were very different to us in that they were very fair skinned, not used to spending long amounts of time outdoors in the strong sun, and not very athletic at all. We didn't end up spending much time with them, but it really was fascinating to meet distant family and share our stories.

After spending two years in Mount Hagen and landing this amazing job that I loved and making some very dear friends, my husband received a job offer on Bougainville Island where the mining industry was absolutely booming. His skills were highly sought after so we made the decision to relocate. It was a sad farewell but life as an expat has an expiry date and there are constant arrivals and farewells, so we knew it was the right decision for us.

Arriving in Arawa I was shocked at the heat and humidity. I found it very difficult to acclimatise to this sudden change in weather patterns, having grown used to the warm days of dry heat and the afternoon thunderstorms bringing rain and very cool nights in the highlands. At one point I didn't think I'd be able to breathe properly again, I found it so difficult to draw a long breath. But as with anything, my body adapted, and we settled into a new location.

Bougainville had so much to offer in the way of water sports and activities. We learned to scuba dive and went out in our newfound friends' boat regularly, diving, swimming and picnicking on nearby beaches. The lifestyle was different but every bit as wonderful as it had been in Mount Hagen.

I also landed a job as soon as I arrived, this time – wait for it – as an internal auditor in the Papua New Guinea Banking Corporation, or PNGBC, an extension of the Commonwealth Bank of Australia. I had absolutely zero experience in a job that was pretty important, but who was I to refuse a challenge?

Again, I learned on the job and soon loved going to work, meeting new people and being challenged in my role, foreign as I was to it. We spent one year in this beautiful location and loved every minute of the adventure. I think that living this lifestyle at such a young age gave me an opportunity to mature quickly in many ways while also enjoying stability in a relationship. My feminine instincts of making a house a home very quickly were nurtured alongside the opportunity to become involved in varied activities and challenges.

We continued our life of socialising and dinner parties, this time with an island feel and lighter food than we had regularly been having in the cooler climate. The exotic range and availability of fruits was mouthwatering and simply divine. New Year's Eve 1985 was memorable, it was to be our last one there unfortunately, and we celebrated with our expat friends, enjoying living a lifestyle that not many others were privy to, in my opinion. By this I mean I feel privileged to have known a lifestyle where you had to go out of your comfort zone to make family in a community of mixed nationalities. I loved the community that was built through the desire to connect, explore and grow.

After only a short time I found aerobics classes which were held in a large community hall. When I first went, I was surprised to see around one hundred people eagerly participating in these classes, held two to three times per week. There was one main instructor, Didi and another one Sandy being trained by Didi.

I loved being able to explore aerobics outside of my living room and was quickly singled out as being instructor material. It wasn't what I was expecting it at all, but I was very honoured and excited and scared to take up the challenge of instructing such an eager and fit group of people, also loving that there were just as many men as there were women. I had been leading a small group of women through the videos when living in Mount Hagen but had never choreographed and created a music playlist to instruct a class from scratch. It took me out of my comfort zone to prepare for this role.

I knew that we were lucky, but I also knew that we were more than just lucky. It was a choice to throw caution to the wind and choose to move away from familiarity, security and of course family and friends, to explore a life a little outside the norms of most people. Things can go wrong, we could have realised we made a terrible mistake, but we were nothing if not risk takers, and I have that incredible man I married at the tender age of 19 to thank for taking me by the hand and leading me into adventure after adventure.

It was during the last few months of our time there that I realised I could no longer ignore the elephant in the room. That elephant was the level of intimacy in our marriage. It had slowly dwindled while we were too busy living a very full life surrounded by other people and always 'doing' outside of our marriage, with very little 'being' inside our marriage.

I had seen the end coming for a while, although I didn't want to admit it to anyone and quite honestly didn't even want to acknowledge it. It had come to my awareness that while I deeply loved the life I lived while I was with him, I was not 'in love' with the man. I know now, I was never truly in love with him, I was totally infatuated with him, I was in awe of him, I was fascinated and constantly enthralled in the life we lived, but there was something missing, something that had never been there.

With time, this was slowly revealed to me, and it was unfair to continue in the marriage once I was certain of this. I was 23. This amazing man had entered my life with a whoosh, swept me off my feet, showed me the world, thrown me into opportunities and adventures I never would have dreamed of – he was my Aladdin and I had been on a magical carpet ride for six years.

I have always believed that people come into your life for a reason, a season or a lifetime. Very rarely do many stay for a lifetime, and my experience is that it's almost always a reason and a season combined. This has allowed me to close chapters of my life when I feel the knowing deep within that it's time to move forward without trying to cling onto something that wasn't meant to be – whether that be an idea, a business, a partnership, friendship, relationship, job or another aspect of life.

Too often there is a clutching onto the past or hanging on for the potential it has. There is absolutely no way that one person can successfully hold a relationship together without the absolute support and desire of the other. It only ends in bitterness, grief and heartbreak when it could have been a parting of ways, taking the blessings or the lessons it brought. It's not always blessings and it's not always amicable, but your life went on that path and that's what there is to work with. No going back, only forward.

In the words of Abraham-Hicks, it's like trying to consistently swim upstream. It's exhausting and eventually you tire, you become exhausted and can't go on. Then there comes the time to feel into the reasons you are in the situation that requires you to go against the flow of your life and perhaps reevaluate things. Or to just drop in exhaustion, and then get up and continue swimming upstream, angry, determined to prove your point, and against your gut instincts. The lessons are always there, the clues are as subtle as a Mack truck but often our hurt and pain and anger override them.

FOUR

SYDNEY LIFE, BABIES AND MARRIAGE

Leaving PNG was something I didn't want to do, I would have loved to stay on working and living there for at least another year, however since I didn't have the working visa, only my husband did, I was not allowed to stay without the correct channels being undertaken and a contract with my place of work being entered into. So, I decided it was time to come home and move forward, beginning with living with Mum and Dad until I sorted out what I was going to do.

During this time back in Wollongong I continued staying in contact with a man I had worked with at the bank, Graeme. There had been chemistry there and he had been a good friend to me when I was going through my separation and making the tough decisions. Our communication became more intense and we decided that when he came home in a few months' time we would see how we fitted together, outside of the environment of Bougainville.

During those months I got a job in Sydney, working in a typing/clerical pool for the Australian Government Solicitors Office in Sydney CBD. I commuted 90 minutes each way by train and worked in that boring and unfulfilling job because it had quite a few benefits. I could get one day off every second week by taking advantage of flex time. I joined a touch footy team and we played in our lunch time once or twice a week in the nearby beautiful playing grounds. I actually enjoyed being in the city and out of Wollongong.

As it turned out, Graeme and I decided to move in together immediately after he arrived back in Sydney. He had a house that had been rented out, so he arranged for the tenants to move out in time for us to move straight in upon his return. It seemed right and also exciting, albeit a very quick decision for such a big move in our long-distance relationship. I guess we both thought we might as well just jump in and see how things go, we certainly had chemistry and my job location was perfect too, a much less time-consuming commute from the north west suburbs of Sydney.

Fast forward three months, and I found out I was pregnant. Not exactly planned but we were ecstatic nonetheless, there wasn't a moment's hesitation about this baby. So, we settled into domestic bliss, and I formed lovely friendships with both of his sisters who were beginning to start their own families and also lived nearby.

When our daughter Angela was born, I became a full-time mum. It was a role I relished, and Graeme fully supported and encouraged me in this decision. By the time I gave up work a few weeks before Angela was born, I was really over office work and had no burning desire to get back to it anyway. I was excited to be with my baby for every defining moment of her development. She was a perfect baby and grew up closely surrounded by her cousins as they were born before and after her, both on my side and on Graeme's side of the family.

When she turned one, I began getting itchy feet, wanting to do something outside of being a full-time mum, but something that wouldn't take me away from home for too long. I wanted it all! So, the synchronicities of the universe came into play, and a beautiful friend of mine, also Carmel, suggested very strongly that I should attain my instructing certification. We had worked together after I came back to Sydney, and in that time, I had also done what I had done in PNG, led lunchtime aerobics classes. Yep, still Jane Fonda. Carmel knew that I would be a good candidate to put my skills to use in the fitness industry.

I resisted, so she dared me to make it my New Year's resolution for 1988/89 – which I did. Back then it was only a nine-day course and that gave me my qualifications to instruct and be a personal trainer. I went on to study Cert III and IV many years later to update my somewhat mediocre personal training qualifications.

I finished the course on a Friday, and quite literally fell into my first teaching job on the following Monday. I was so unprepared, but my new boss wasn't going to take any excuses, so I had to mix a tape and put together my own choreography for a one hour class. To say I was nervous beyond reason is an understatement. When I taught that first class to a room of about 20 women at 9.30 on a Monday morning, my stomach was doing backflips. I was so scared I would freeze, forget the moves and sequences and just completely fuck it up.

After the warm up I got them into a movement pattern and then ran out of the room without warning, racing to the bathroom just in time – I won't go into details – and then raced back to casually join in and teach the class again. I made it through, no one threw things at me or complained, so I had passed my test. Phew! In the 80s those morning women were a force to be reckoned with, so if you got their approval, you were very happy.

During the following two years I went on to work at several gyms in the area, at one stage I had classes at five different venues and absolutely loved the lifestyle. I was doing something I loved and was being an encouraging role model to other women, I earned some money, made some lifelong friends, met so many incredible people (and still do), I got to be with my daughter almost all the time, and she benefitted by the social interactions with the other children in the crèche when I was teaching. We were all happy and had begun really settling into being a family.

I loved my life and my little family. We had lots of social gatherings with both sides of our families, but Graeme and I began having some issues in our relationship. It didn't seem like anything that we couldn't work through. Well, in hindsight we could have worked through them better if our communication skills had been stronger and if I hadn't felt like I could fix our problems by myself.

The challenges became more and more difficult for me to cope with and I felt hopeless to stand up to my partner who was having some deep personal issues and refused to acknowledge his more frequent bitter moods and abhorrent behaviour. We didn't have the tools to move through this, so I tried my best to rise above my emotions but was really bottling them up. He went in and out of his dark phases and silent periods. It was torture getting through some of those days not knowing what I had said or done to make him not speak to me and totally ignore me. Of course, I know now that it wasn't me, but when you're deep in the spiral of pain and a victim of your own lack of healthy boundaries and standards, it's easy to fall into the belief that you are the one to blame in some way.

I even had a short-lived affair during this period. It happened without warning when I was in an emotionally vulnerable state. We had been invited to a friend's birthday party and were looking forward to it, even lined up my in-laws to babysit. Then when it was time to get ready to go out Graeme announced he didn't want to go any more. Now these were very close, dear friends of ours and we had known about the party for several weeks, so I really wanted to go and celebrate with them. I couldn't convince him to go, so while he called his parents to tell them not to come and babysit, I went on my own, leaving him to sulk in his mood.

At the party, while standing on my own, a very charismatic, handsome and charming man introduced himself to me and we talked for a while. He knew who I was through our friends, and I talked about my husband and daughter. He was also married. When I was waiting for a taxi home, he noticed I was leaving and waited outside with me, where he really laid on the charm, he made me feel beautiful and desired with his smooth talk – something I hadn't felt or heard for quite some time from my husband.

The affair was short lived and involved lots of alcohol. He would sometimes call my home when he was drunk and wasted, telling me he loved me but conveniently didn't remember the next day. I didn't know at the time, but he had a very expensive cocaine habit and party lifestyle which his executive banking salary afforded him easily. Over the years I've read a lot about the psychology around affairs and it definitely holds true for me that it was NOT about the sex. In fact, the sex was extremely disappointing and drunkenly clumsy. It was all about being seen and appreciated after living in the absence of affection for too long. I felt sexy and desired, and – particularly for a Taurus woman – the need for that is as important as oxygen in a relationship.

It transpired that the stress and anxiety of having this huge and shameful secret was definitely not what I wanted in my life. I was using it as an escape and when I acknowledged that, it was a relief to let it go and take another look at my life. I realised that I wanted to turn things around in my relationship if that was possible and so chose to be completely present without the distraction of a toxic situation. With a fresh dose of guilt now sitting firmly inside me, I made a deal with the devil – or God, I'm not sure which one – to keep my secret in exchange for me being unwaveringly committed to my relationship and my family.

Over the coming months I became devoted to giving everything to my little family without the distraction I had created, and life became wonderful once again. I loved being a mother and definitely wanted more than one child, so I thought it was time to have another baby. Graeme agreed, and I was pregnant again quite quickly after that. I honestly thought we would be together forever, especially since I was on my best behaviour to repent for my sins, feeling like I had been given another chance to really appreciate what I had. To stop sabotaging my life by listening to the voices telling me I was unfulfilled, to keep that vault sealed so that I wouldn't let anyone down ever again. All I had to do was rise above our problems, surely that was possible with time.

Things went pretty smoothly again for quite some time between us, and we even got married the year after Emily was born. By the time she was two we really began knowing we had bigger problems than we had been acknowledging. Our communication had not improved as time went on and we were both often miserable and frustrated with each other. I began living with another new companion, anxiety, and dermatitis started coming up on my hands and arms in response to the inner stifled emotions I chose to carry.

We went to marriage counseling and tried to bring some of those suggestions into our relationship, which worked for a little while until old patterns and habits just rose again and again. We both continued getting weighed down in our own silent worlds, each being misunderstood by the other. By Christmas 1993 it was the beginning of the end of our almost eight years together. As I told Graeme, it was like my heart had been shattered into a million pieces and I couldn't find all those pieces anymore. I know he felt this too, and he gave his all in the coming months to create a loving home for the girls to spend time with him. No separation is without pain, regardless of the reason, and I'm proud of all of us for having grown through this individually and together as lovingly as we knew how.

Graeme has always remained a very active and constant figure in the girls' lives. From the beginning, being an avid camper, we had many camping adventures, many of them being with other families we came to know through the squash competitions we played, as well as with my sisters and brothers in law and their families. They were always great trips and adventures, and the girls were fortunate to explore so much outside of suburban life. To this day they both love camping and do so with their husbands when they can.

During the years after the divorce, the girls travelled all over Australia on camping trips with Graeme and his four-wheel driving groups, often up to six weeks long. Bush camping is in their nature now, they can put up a tent in no time, make a camp fire, cook a meal – all of the things they were taught practically from those very early years. They now go exploring national parks with their husbands, often finding incredible places to stay and camp for a weekend or more and have encouraged their friends to join in on the camping life many times.

Years ago, after one long trip away, the girls and I were driving to visit my parents in Wollongong which is about a 90-minute trip. They needed to use the bathroom, so I told them to wait until the next place there was a bathroom. They said to not worry about that, just stop and they would go in the bushes. So I stopped on the long stretch of country road we were on, out they got and did their thing, obviously still used to the outback bush toilet system.

I love that they have had him in their lives so practically, he really has been and continues to be an incredible father and role model, despite the things he comes out with that we roll our eyes at! He has never treated them like precious princesses, rather he taught them to get their hands dirty and participate in life fully wherever possible. These experiences have shaped the girls lives forever in a very positive way. They are adventurous and confident, never afraid of a challenge and are both now blissfully married and expecting their first babies within a few months of each other.

FIVE

THE YEARS WITH MY GIRLS

Being a single mother was something I had never factored into my life and I was really scared to be alone with my daughters. I had never been alone before in my life. I went from living with my parents, to living with Greg in another country, back to Mum and Dad, then straight into living with Graeme. In the weeks following our separation I could hardly sleep at night, hearing imaginary noises and being spooked at my own thoughts.

My recurring nightmare as I laid in a restless sleep with total fear-paralyses was that a murderous intruder had just broken into the house, made his way to Angela's bedroom where he murdered her, then Emily's bedroom where he murdered her and then was just outside my door waiting to finish the slaying. We had to sell the house to complete settlement and so I had a choice to make. I had the option to move back to Wollongong and stay with Mum until I sorted out what I was going to do. It would be a safe option; I would be surrounded by family and there wouldn't be as much pressure on me to support the three of us.

But I also had the life that I had built over the last eight years and it was a life I loved. The girls all had so many beautiful friendships here, they were now turning seven and four. As well as being close to Graeme which would make life much easier for shared custody, my sisters in law were here with their children, and the cousins were all so close. There was too much swaying me to stay in the area, not the least being my work and the friendships I had formed through my work. I had created an incredible lifestyle with my career in the fitness industry, and the opportunities I had in Sydney would have been nonexistent in Wollongong. So, the decision was made, we would stay put and rent a place for us to call home.

The girls and I blossomed throughout these years together. They had what seemed to be the perfect balance possible after a divorce. Initially there were separation issues which were heartbreaking to watch, but we got through those times knowing there was no turning back, no matter how much we missed the family unit. I was able to support us financially with no problem since I had added to my income stream by making fitness apparel. It began just with me making my own workout gear, so that I could have lots of outfits without spending a fortune and ended up with me growing that into a small business.

I converted the single garage into a production room. I bought a secondhand boardroom table, which was my cutting table, got a second hand industrial overlocker on eBay, and an industrial straight sewing machine, again second hand. I'm a great shopper, so ended up with an efficient setup where I would create and make tights, leotards, crop tops and running shorts. My label was Bodyshock, and I had labels made up to sew onto the items, I took pride in my work and loved that I could add another way to earn while not having to leave our home. Since I was working at several locations, I wasn't short of customers and they literally got made to measure workout gear. I remained small, choosing not to employ anyone else since I didn't feel I had the resources or the skills to market and grow the business.

There was internal access from my workroom to the house, so I was always very close to the girls when I was working. They would wander in and out and Emily would always be writing me beautiful little love notes and would deliver them to me while I cut and sewed away. Often, they would dress in the outfits I made for them and put on my aerobics music and play instructor, taking turns to each be the aerobics instructor and the participant. I loved watching them mimic me, I wish I had taken videos and photos of them, it was too cute and such great memories to have for all of us.

I also started dating someone I met at one of the health clubs I worked at, and this became a relationship that allowed us both to introduce our children. We had great times as an extended family group with his kids, as well as lots of fun and intimacy as a couple when our children were with their respective other parent. After just over two years though, I found out he had been seeing someone else for a year, and I was devastated. I gave him a second chance, and he proved unable to stay loyal to me, so I ended it immediately upon finding this out.

I was pretty shattered; I'd never had my trust in someone broken like this before. I just didn't get it – why wouldn't he just break up with me and date her? We weren't living together or engaged, but I had been under the impression we were exclusive and may have eventually headed down that track. Maybe it was karma, but it definitely didn't feel nice, and it made me vulnerable to jealousy, as I was about to find out.

SIX

ANDREW, MARRIAGE AND BUSINESS

Music was and is an essential component to group exercise, and in 1996 we were either mixing our own tapes or purchasing pre-mixed tapes from new emerging companies taking advantage of this need in the industry. I became a distributor for Trax music and made a small commission selling and delivering their music to fellow instructors. I had a pretty good customer base and it added to my income stream, all within the same industry.

One of the gyms I worked at had just been sold, and I met the new owner one day as I was dropping off an order for an instructor friend. We got chatting and he was a bit flirty, as was I since I was now newly single again. He asked me out, and I said no the first couple of times, only because my old boyfriend was still contacting me and even though it was over, I didn't want him to find out I was dating someone new just yet. Then I decided to not be held to ransom by my ex's ego and childish behaviour, and just go out with this new guy since it wasn't fair that my life should be put on hold, and I was the one doing that.

And so began a wonderful love story with Andrew. He had just purchased his first business after retiring from a professional athletics career due to chronic injury. In the first year we dated he received a business proposal to establish a health club within a very large social club, and he won this hands down with his incredible ideas and projections. Being a born entrepreneur and ideas man, this was a dream come true, and before long the new club was established and was fast becoming the most popular and successful health club in the area.

It was like a dream, his business was going really well, and our relationship was also blossoming. My girls loved him, and we spent a lot of time together as a family when they were with me, and had our couple time when they were with Graeme. Even though the business was taking off during this time, there was a lot of debt too, so we never really had a lot of money. That actually made life more interesting though, seeing what we could do, what adventures we could go on, on a tight budget. Picnics were a favourite, and we would take our little dogs Georgie and Lucy – miniature chihuahua sisters which we had bought for the girls' birthdays – to our favourite place by the river on many Sundays. There were also countless road trips to Wollongong and Canberra visiting our parents and often staying the weekend.

We did hit a few hurdles though. One of the major ones happened after we began living together in my home, and it resulted in him moving out for several weeks. It began when I was triggered continually by Andrew going out every few weeks with his mates, or even with one friend. I actually loved that he had strong friendships and nurtured them, but the green-eyed monster of jealousy raised its ugly head, and I became resentful of him going out. I fought this feeling with all I had, but that didn't stop my instinctual behaviour whenever he said he would be going out. That's when the silent treatment would begin and I felt a different persona come over me, one that I desperately did not want to be in. My entire personality shifted, and it was so obvious that I was behaving in a childish way. Waves of jealousy went through me and my thoughts spiraled out of control in all the 'what-if' scenarios. What if he met someone? What if he cheated on me, it's happened before?'

Eventually he told me he wouldn't stay if I continued that way, since he hadn't done, nor was he even thinking of doing anything that I should be jealous of or threatened by. He moved out and it was awful, I really didn't want him to go but he knew it wasn't going to work if I didn't trust him.

During those weeks I began swimming, I continued running, the girls and I had fun on our weekend trips to Wollongong visiting family, the girl's dancing and swimming lessons continued. I found out that I was feeling so free, and I didn't even try to do anything to change anything about me or my behaviour. I just let go of anything that didn't bring happiness into my life. It was crazy how great I felt when I thought I'd be miserable and really missing Andrew.

After those couple of months apart, Andrew asked if a friend of his visiting from Canada could stay at my place since his accommodation had fallen through. I told him no, I wasn't going to have this friend staying with me, not unless Andrew was moving back in. And that I wasn't interested in him moving back in unless it was for all the right reasons, meaning unless it was that we were getting back together.

So, the friend stayed, Andrew moved back in and for some reason, I never became jealous of him again. A shift had occurred, and I wasn't sure how or when, but that didn't matter to me, I was so happy that we were back together. In hindsight I had stepped up in my self confidence and self empowerment and let go of the jealousies and insecurities I had carried over with me from the last relationship. The worst had happened, I had pushed Andrew away and then had to continue living without a supportive man in my life. But I hadn't crumbled. I didn't have nightmares. In fact, it was the opposite and even though I didn't understand what had happened, I forged ahead with a newfound confidence and outlook on life.

Three years into our relationship, he proposed to me while on holiday in Bali. We planned our wedding for just three months later. One reason for a short engagement was that we planned to have at least one child together, and I was in my mid-thirties – he was five years younger – and my biological clock was ticking. The wedding was perfect, held in the Southern Highlands in November. We had the ceremony in a tiny old sandstone church, and the reception at a beautifully restored bed and breakfast. Both girls were junior bridesmaids, if that's even a thing but they were too old to be flower girls and not quite old enough to be bridesmaids. I made their dresses, Mum arranged the flowers and bouquets which were stunning, she's a retired florist, and the day went perfectly, with Dad walking me down the aisle. He was pretty good at it now!

We had a surprise guest at our wedding, but he was hardly noticed, in fact, he was our big secret. I was six weeks pregnant with Ryan. I hadn't been trying to fall pregnant and was even on the pill, although my pill taking regime probably wasn't on point, but that sure took away the pressure of actively waiting to get pregnant. I had to pretend to take sips of champagne the whole evening which was a little awkward.

Unbeknown to us, a small group of friends were taking some social drugs at the reception, which would have been neither here nor there, if it hadn't been for one of the guests, a work colleague of Andrew's who had been taking something, becoming quite emotional and upset.

The host of the B&B approached me to come and talk to this woman, but when I found out who it was, I knew it was Andrew who should be talking to her. I knew she didn't like me, even though I wasn't sure why since I couldn't think of anything I'd done to upset her over the last few years we had known each other; she was just always aloof around me. Andrew went and settled her down, and by that stage the reception was ending, and I had gone to our room upstairs.

When he came in, I asked him if she was okay, and what he told me came as a surprise. He said that she asked him if he tried calling her a couple of months ago and left a message. He told her he didn't but apparently, she liked him, and had really liked him for some time – and this was obviously the reason she didn't like me. I knew they carried on at work having fun and jokes, but that's all it was. When she received that message that she thought he had left her on her answering machine many months before, she was under the impression he was interested in her. Now this was all going on in her head, but here she was as an invited guest to our wedding, having a humiliating meltdown and asking if he was really sure he wanted to marry me. I did feel for her, it must have been tormenting, but the drugs didn't help, and it was probably not the time to be asking the groom if he was sure about his choice of bride!

Andrew was the instigator of the incredible relationship in our extended family, particularly with Graeme. Early on in our relationship, Andrew would spend a lot of time with the three of us. When Graeme came to pick up the girls for the weekend, he would usually wait at the door for the girls to come out, and they would leave after kissing us goodbye. One Saturday morning was different though. Before Graeme arrived, Andrew said he wanted to let any grievances between the two of them be put in the past. If we were going to move forward in our relationship, and it looked like we were heading to a long future together, then it would be so much better for all involved to move past any friction.

And so, when Graeme arrived, Andrew answered the door, shook his hand and invited him in for a cuppa. Crickets! I remember Graeme being caught off guard for a moment before accepting and then coming inside to join us as we then sat down and chatted. Since that day, we have all grown closer as an extended family, and this has made family occasions not only less uncomfortable, but enjoyable and so much more amazing. Imagine the love being shared around stepbrothers and sisters, with the parents and their new partners all sincerely enjoying each other's company.

This evolved to many Christmas celebrations at my ex in-laws' homes where we were accepted with open arms as our family had expanded with our two sons, Ryan and Daniel. I truly love my entire family, the extended one that has been created and forged and blended over the past 23 years. Celebrating my daughters' engagements and weddings this last year is the culmination of years of acceptance, forgiveness and unconditional love.

SEVEN

THE BUSINESS JOURNEY

Andrew's company grew quickly after that. The first acquisition was a popular and established health club very close by. It had a large membership base and enormous potential. Until only months before, I had been working at that club instructing for several years, so I had a good relationship with both the owner and many of the instructors. In fact, the reason I resigned was because working at both clubs was contradictory to the forward momentum of our own business. It was like working for the enemy, and although instructors have the freedom to freelance regardless of location, I agreed that I would remain loyal to our brand.

One morning we heard that members of this club were unable to enter. All doors were locked and there was a notice on the entrance saying it had closed. No warning, no explanation. Andrew immediately saw the opportunity, one where, if the owner agreed, the members could remain at their beloved club and have their membership fees honoured. We got in contact with the owner and arranged a meeting for the following day. The result of that meeting was that Andrew acquired the membership base at a price that was a bargain for what he had in mind, whilst also allowing the owner to walk away with money in his pocket instead of zilch. Lawyers made the sale legal and the lease was taken over. An iconic health club had been saved and would soon undergo a big facelift.

Most of the staff remained as well as a whole new team of sales staff and a manager. In no time there was a healthy growth which meant that long overdue renovations could be undertaken. Designers and decorators were employed and collaborated with, and by the time the renovations were complete it was 'the' place to be, drawing young mums with a state of the art child care centre, play land with giant slides and jumping castles that their children didn't want to leave. The latest technology in gym floor and cardio equipment was purchased, and the best group fitness timetable around meant that the classes were filled to capacity on a regular basis, in a room that held up to 120 participants.

This enormous success in such a short period of time was a primer into more acquisitions. Only a couple of the following ones were not always well thought out and ended up bringing a tonne of bad debt with them. I understand that sometimes the opportunity and the potential can be heady and deem the downside almost invisible and secondary when compared to the possibilities – but they were overlooked nonetheless when they should have been a big warning sign. At the height of the company there were a total of eight health clubs in Sydney. The ones that were performing profitably were incredibly well-oiled machines which ran smoothly, but the ones which were acquired with accompanying debt were quickly and dangerously draining the profits of the ones without that burden of old debt.

One of the main clubs had all onsite parking, as well as street parking taken away by the local Council due to a planning change in the area. Then a Fitness First club opened up very close by within a Westfield Shopping Centre, hence plenty of parking, and they brazenly put their salespeople outside our front door to solicit our members. In the blink of an eye, what was a profitable and growing club turned into one losing members by the day. Then began a long slow spiral downwards into financial difficulty.

It was the expansion of our business, and then the decline into eventual administration and bankruptcy that took us on the wildest and most destructive ride of our lives. Ego definitely ruled the day with much of the business expansion during the previous few years. However there was never any ill intention on Andrew's part. In fact, the very opposite, so during the inevitable slippery slide into the final months, weeks and days of trading, every effort possible was made to look after staff and creditors. This unfortunately wasn't as it was seen, with many bitter staff throwing wild accusations and personal attacks on my husband, and sometimes me too when they didn't receive all of their entitlements.

I completely understood their grievances but there was nothing we could do at that stage. We had borrowed money, quite a substantial amount, from my husband's parents to help save the company, and had received money from two other investors, and this too was lost. We lost our home, our cars and literally everything we had other than our personal belongings. And since we had not been taking proper wages or paying into our superannuation for a long time, this didn't exactly add up to much.

Depression and anxiety were our newest companions at that time, and it was distressing living each day at the peril of the administrators, in fear of our future, being stripped of so much on every level.

There were visits to the lawyer's office which I attended as well, so as to understand firsthand the next steps and our options moving forward. These meetings were some of the most gut-wrenching moments of my life. There is one other time which I will mention later in the book, however in these moments which seemed to last eternally, I held back torrents of waves of emotions that had been building for many, many months. I felt so powerless, so angry and I was grieving so deeply, all at the same time. I knew something big was ending and our lives would not be the same, but I didn't realise the potential I held in directing the outcome. Instead I didn't let the wall break down. I held it all in and became withdrawn, and in those meetings, I literally couldn't speak for fear of falling into a psychotic heap of uncontrollable wailing right there on the floor. That was not an option, so I allowed some persistent tears to silently escape, belying the cacophony that lie beneath them, and stopped talking, held it in, and sat there like a ghost of myself.

I felt like I was failing in every area of my life. My health, my marriage, being a good mother and being there for my children, and I was definitely not in a good place with my relationship with myself.

I relay this story in some detail to highlight the despair I had fallen into, along with a feeling of helplessness and powerlessness. I felt defeated. But life had to go on. We moved into a three-bedroom rental property, which meant that the girls would need to share a bedroom now after having their own rooms for the previous three years, but the bonus was we had a pool and this lovely old home felt warm and it held us together for the following three years. We had some incredible times together there and took steps forward, then steps back. I took control of most of our finances in paying off school fee debts and tax office payments, along with all the household bills which was enriching and empowering for me. It also allowed Andrew to begin the journey into rebuilding his career.

In this time, I studied and attained my Certificate III and IV in Personal Training and Group Fitness as Andrew worked tirelessly at building once again from scratch while dealing with his own emotional fallout. But we did it together and that was a very healing and restorative time for us as a family. The enormous pressure of the business was off, and even though our family was still reeling from damaged relationships on another level, we did the best we could. We moved to a new house again in 2010.

EIGHT
TRIATHLON

Triathlon played a significant role in my life. It allowed me so much freedom and self-expression. I discovered talents I wasn't aware I had, and it opened up a whole new avenue where I formed friendships that were life changing.

As with most of the life changing chapters of my life, I didn't go searching for it, it found me. I had taken up running when I met Andrew in 1996. He was a recently retired world class athlete, his event had been the 400 metre hurdles no less – a demanding and brutal event at that level, and he still enjoyed staying fit since his retirement through injury.

I'll always remember my first run back then. We were meeting for lunch, but he was delayed and I was early, so he suggested I go for a run while I was waiting for him. I know this sounds weird, but the meeting place was at his gym and I was in my training gear. I went off into the back streets and got a bit lost and ended up running a few more kilometres than expected. It was tough but invigorating and as with all exercise I performed, I felt great afterwards for having done it. After that, running became a part of my fitness routine once more, for the first time since the days in PNG which was 10 years prior.

When our son Ryan was born in 2000 it wasn't long before I wanted to begin a light training regime. I was shopping for a new pair of running shoes and asked the guy in the Athlete's Foot store for any information on local running groups I could join. He gave me the number of Bruce Thomas, an Australian Ironman legend, but I didn't know that at the time. I called Bruce, who happened to be married to another athlete and an instructor I worked with at a fitness centre a few years prior. With no knowledge of who he was, I agreed to meet him at the local pool, Waves Aquatic Centre where he was coaching a swim squad session. I took my swimming costume and goggles and joined in the slow lane to have a swim and then have a chat afterwards about the running group he spoke about.

As it turned out, I loved being in the water again. I had learned from a good friend the art of effective swimming techniques when I was around 20 and training for my bronze surfing medallion. It felt great to be moving through the water once more. So, after our chat, I realised he was a triathlon coach – still had no idea of his legendary status – and joined him in swim squads and track running sessions on a regular basis.

Being around triathletes in these sessions, it was hard not to be intrigued in the sport of triathlon, so I thought I'd buy a bike and see if I enjoyed riding. I used to cycle to and from work when I lived in Wollongong quite often so was no stranger to it but hadn't done any real distance training. My brother Tim, a triathlete himself warned me against purchasing a new bike since he knew so many people who spent a lot of money on a bike, they used only a few times. He loaned me a spare road bike he had, and I trained on that.

Within a few months I competed in my first enticer triathlon, a distance of 250 metre swim, 10 kilometre bike ride and 2.5 kilometre run. I loved it. The feeling of exhaustion closely followed by elation after the race, then taking out third place in my age group and taking home a small trophy left me on top of the world. I couldn't wait to race again. My cool down after the race was breastfeeding my four-month-old son! I loved that my family was there cheering me on.

I joined the Hills Triathlon Club and quickly formed some new friends and training buddies. Initially I began competing in some smaller sprint distance races – 500 metre swim, 20 kilometre ride and 5 kilometre run – at Kurnell in Sydney's south. Then I felt a desire to test the waters, and the fitness levels on the Olympic distance race of 1500 metre swim, 40 kilometre ride and 10 kilometre run. By this time, I had upgraded my road bike, mainly because there had been a few mishaps during races with the chain falling off during the race. I spent precious time stopping to fix the chain a few times in each race, so I guess in a way I was also learning bike maintenance.

Having decided to turn desire into action and challenge myself further, I hired a coach to write me a program that would make me accountable to my training. I was doing well, often placing in the top three in races all over the state and was pleasantly surprised to find I had qualified for the World Triathlon Age Group competition. It was to be held in Cancun Mexico in November 2002. That's when I decided to become serious with my commitment to improving, hence hiring my coach.

This is what my training program looked like. I had one or two training sessions each day, with one rest day per week. Monday, Wednesday and Friday, I always swam in the tri squad, often with Emily. Emily was also a budding triathlete and went on to compete in club and school triathlons with excellent results. She was very talented in the sport too, her strongest leg being the swim, closely followed by the bike (she was a natural in the water) from 5.15–7.00am and covered 5 kilometres in each session. Our swim coach Troy gave us sessions to align with our race schedule with focus on different areas. Our upper body strength and stroke correction training involved using paddles strapped on our hands and bands to bind our ankles together to prevent any kicking. Short fins were used with a paddle board to develop our kick strength and technique. Breathing was improved by swimming laps building our breath intake rate, starting with three-stroke breathing i.e. a breath on every third stroke, then accumulating in twos until we reached nine-stroke breathing, while still holding our technique.

It required so much focus and discipline, yet it was something I really looked forward to. The social component and the camaraderie was special. While we trained hard in the pool, the change rooms were a different story. Alli, Jodie, and I talked and shared so much with each other and became very close. Emily thought we were all weirdos because we didn't care that we were naked or in our underwear in an open change room laughing and chatting after showering. But that's a huge component of sport, the relationships you build along the way. I wouldn't have accomplished what I have if it wasn't for those friendships which went way beyond the pool.

For the running component my program included one track session per week, again building strength, speed and endurance. Now that I was doing Olympic distance my programs sometimes accumulated weekly, for example on the first week I did 6 x 400 metres, leaving on two minutes, meaning regardless of the time I did, I had to begin the next lap of 400 metres right on two minutes.

Each week the number of reps increased by two, so by the fourth week I had to do 12 x 400's leaving on two minutes. It was brutal but it improved my fitness and endurance enormously.

As well as track, I had another three runs including a long slow run on Sundays, increasing in distance over the program. My longest training run on the program for the Olympic distance race (10 kilometre) was 20 kilometres. Always striving to be able to easily accomplish the race distance by training for longer distances and working on the mechanics of movement in the track sessions. My running buddies Alli and Jodie rocked up to my house each Monday afternoon so we could all smash out our long run together, chatting away the miles which melted away behind us. When we got home, Emily was often waiting with a platter of fresh fruit for replenishment, she was always so eager to encourage and support us. Angela and Emily often minded the boys while I went on runs, I don't know how I could have accomplished what I did without their loving and unconditional support.

The training bike rides varied. I did one road ride alone during the week, and one speed or strength session on the wind trainer, a device you place the back wheel into so that you can remain stationary while going through the gears. The program dictated how many minutes to remain in each gear and whether to stay in the saddle (seated) or not. We often did these at my coaches home in a small group which was much more fun.

Sunday was long ride day. Regardless of fitness level, our tri club had an organised ride which usually left at around 6 am, depending on the time of year – earlier in the summer and later in the winter because of the light.

The longest ride for me was 120 kilometres. These rides weren't about speed, but about distance and endurance. The coffee stop on the way back was always the highlight of the morning – again, the social aspect being of extremely high importance for all of us. Sometimes we rode out to a place where we could do hill repeats which were gruelling. Bobbin Head was one of those places we did hills. I'm talking long winding roads with steady climbs where the aim was to stay in the saddle all the way to the top which was a couple of kilometres, then spinning on the way down rather than not using your legs at all, always keeping the legs turning over.

Alli, Jodie and I all raced in Cancun after each qualifying for a spot in our age groups, and had an absolute blast experiencing the huge international event that it was. We had arranged a fund-raising evening to assist with our trip and were successful in raising enough to cover the entire trip, which was great for me since it didn't put a strain on our finances.

After the racing was over, we had a few days to sight-see the beautiful surroundings, and then it was home to our families. We all continued on with our training during the off season so that by the time we were racing again we all qualified once more for the World's in New Zealand. I had just fallen pregnant with my fourth baby when I was racing my last qualifying race in Mooloolaba, in which I placed third, so had to decline the championships since I would be eight months pregnant on race day.

Once Daniel was born in November 2003, I slowly got back into the swing of training again. Stronger than ever because I had a good fitness base, I once again qualified, this time for Honolulu in November 2005. I was now being coached by Christina Thomas, Bruce's wife and my old instructor friend who was an elite athlete and former Ironman Champion herself.

It was one evening after a grueling hill run session that she asked if I was feeling okay. We were all stretching and cooling down at the time and I remember being a little surprised at her question since I was feeling great, tired but great. She said that I looked pale and she strongly suggested I have a blood test to check my iron levels. I agreed and made an appointment the following week. When the test results came in, I was again surprised to hear that my iron levels were way below par. I was indeed anaemic, not by a little, by a lot! My ferritin levels were so low there was no reading available of them.

I don't know if it was the knowledge that my results indicated I was anaemic, or if it was just the pinnacle moment of my body responding to the lack of oxygen getting to my energy systems after fighting to perform, but the next run I went on I had to stop in exhaustion after just 100 metres. I literally wanted to collapse, and simply couldn't go on.

This was six weeks out from Worlds in Honolulu, and I was devastated yet determined to compete no matter what. Under coaches and doctors' orders I trained very little in the weeks leading up to the race. I had a store of training under my belt that would hopefully get me through on race day. During this time, I had some iron injections but reacted badly so couldn't rely on having more. I had to rely on my dietary intake which was so hard for me.

Race day finally came, and I competed. I made it through the swim, and the bike ride and when it came to the 10km run I didn't know if I could do it. I made a pact with myself that at each drink station, which were at one-kilometre intervals around the course, I would allow myself to walk for a bit. This mind game got me through, and I eventually ran down the finish chute, depleted but happy.

When I got home, I stopped all training and tried to recover. As it turns out it would take ten years before I would finally be showing normal blood test results with regards to iron levels again.

It was unfortunate on a few levels, one of which I wish I could change. Emily had been training with me consistently for many months leading up to the race in many sessions and was so excited for the race. She really wanted to come and support me and the team, but it just wasn't financially viable.

For both of the international races the girls and I held fundraisers, to raise all the money we needed to travel, stay, and compete. We profited enough to cover the trip 100%. Andrew's company was not doing well enough to support anything other than our immediate commitments and there were no savings, so I couldn't take my daughter.

Sadly, after I returned and wasn't up to any of my regular training schedule, she also stopped training and competing.

In hindsight I would go back and support her training as much as she had supported mine, so she could go on to compete in more races, the ones outside school, like I had been competing in.

Hindsight is a wonderful thing though.

NINE
STRENGTH TRAINING AND BODY SHAPING

In the forced downtime I stumbled across something I had never before considered. I was having lunch with a good friend from my early instructing years, Lea. As we were enjoying our get together, I noticed some girls looking very tanned, with faces and hair done beautifully, at the cafe. Lea pointed out that there must be a body building competition upstairs in the Club. I looked at the girls, admiring their dedication to training and diet, and their sheer guts to get up there on stage and compete. As we were talking, I asked Lea, do you think I could ever do something like that? Well, she jumped at the comment and said that she would like to take my 'skinned rabbit' looking body and put some muscle on it, and yes it would not only be possible, but she would train me.

Lea was a long-time body builder and had competed over many years, and trained clients to do the same. So, with my trainer lined up, she took me through my program and set out my training schedule. It was only three times per week and began with basic moves including squats, deadlifts, bench press, shoulder and arm work, mostly all on machines since I was an amateur and needed to build my base and technique before doing free weights. For the first few months each session included all body parts, and then Lea began breaking the program down to legs, shoulders and abs, back and arms.

I could handle this type of training since it was short and sharp. We began training and met once a week at the gym, and I worked the program by myself another two to three days a week. Before long I began noticing improvements and muscle gain. It wasn't long before I was looking at entering my first competition. Within a year of beginning a weight training program I was on stage, fake tan, ridiculously high heels, half-starved and performing a little routine for the judges. I took home a trophy for second place. This wasn't too difficult since there were usually only a handful of competitors in each age group, and in my first competition there were three of us in my category.

I competed for two years before hanging up my bikini and heels. It was time to focus on gaining my personal training qualification so I could run some programs in one of Andrew's health clubs. The programs I took clients through once I had my qualification were 12-week lifestyle programs. I loved seeing the results during the three-month journey so many clients undertook. Them trusting me to be there for them not only in the capacity as trainer, but to support them emotionally and mentally was wonderful.

I learned very quickly that behind excess body fat is often sadness, loneliness, unhappiness, abandonment, guilt, shame, and a veritable cocktail of unresolved emotions. I knew that I had used food as a source of power as a teenager and understood that often food is seen as the only power we have. We can use it to satiate our emotions, to quieten inner voices craving acceptance, to slowly poison our system, to shape us into acceptable forms to please someone else, or to avoid being seen, or being available. So many options are available for us to overlook the basic role of food as our source of nourishment and health and to abuse it for our own distorted cravings.

Even though I was teaching others how to eat to nourish and thrive, how to exercise to become strong, to beat diseases and conditions that had them thinking they had a death sentence, I was still way below the iron levels I should have been at. I was avoiding looking after myself, and I couldn't understand why I was doing this. Yes, I was eating healthy, but I wasn't doing anything to improve my iron levels from the drastically low level they had been on for a couple of years. Something inside me avoided taking my iron supplements and eating an abundance of iron rich foods. I even drank coffee and tea knowing it would inhibit the absorption of the iron I so desperately needed. I wanted to be healthy again, but I was also sabotaging myself.

Then the next symptom of my emotional sinkhole showed itself. I had been experiencing bleeding gums intermittently for a few years and had also had a period of time when my breath was disgusting, and I was so aware and embarrassed about that. A long overdue visit to the dentist revealed that I had gum disease, and I needed to get myself to a specialist as soon as possible, like yesterday. I booked in to see a periodontist and was quickly diagnosed that this silent disease was spreading very quickly. It had already eaten into the gum surrounding all four of my wisdom teeth and I had receding gums beginning around other teeth. I was booked in to have all my wisdom teeth removed, to avoid the spread of the rampant silent disease and this would hopefully save the rest of my teeth. I then went on to visit my dentist and periodontist alternately and followed my teeth and gum cleaning routine diligently.

So here was my second significant health message. My body was going to keep speaking loudly to me until I finally did something about facing the buried emotional trauma and depression, I was internalising. It was difficult to finally do this since I didn't want to disrupt my life by creating difficult conversations and speaking my truth. But the time had definitely come. I wasn't being the mother I wanted to be, I wasn't there for them emotionally like I should have been and like I wanted to be, I just couldn't cope with any more emotional requirements on my already tired mind and body. Feeling shame and failure as a mother just added to the depression. I had run away so many times from facing not only my own needs, but those of the dearest ones to me, my children.

It was time. It was definitely time.

I began looking into the clues that my body had been giving me in the form of dis-ease. The results of my research told me a story that felt like it had been written just for me, by someone who had been living alongside me for years.

> Anaemia: In metaphysics, blood represents the love of life. Being anaemic means the person has lost this love of life. There is often a feeling that a parasitic person or circumstance that is beyond

your control has drained your life force out of you. Exhausting or traumatic circumstances have been experienced and you can't figure out how to process them. Feeling constantly in fight or flight mode takes a toll emotionally, mentally and physically.

Gum Disease: 1: Gingivitis (bleeding gums) Anger arising with regard to what you can or cannot say. There is regret around not saying what needed to be said in the past, as you know it would have changed the outcome of stressful circumstances that have since taken place. Communication is difficult because you feel challenged to communicate your self-worth and personal opinion.

Gum Disease: 2: Feeling suppressed or threatened by an influential person or partner. Anger and resentment related to making decisions and expressing yourself. Undecided about your feelings about your life circumstances and the people in your life. Feeling frustrated about being indecisive. There is often a partner who is more dominant in the decision-making process.

No wonder I had been feeling resistance in healing my body of its iron deficiency. I was not ready to stand up for my truth or to raise debate around subjects that were intricately woven in our family. For years, I had allowed my daughters to be raised without offering my opinion when it mattered the most. When they were in need of my input the most, in their difficult teenage years, I allowed myself to be convinced that the outcomes and consequences offered by my husband were what was best. It was a convenient way for me to escape responsibility and consequence, and difficult conversations regarding discipline. When the girls and I had been living on our own it was so easy, and they respected my rules and boundaries. But since they now had a stepfather, I could avoid being the strict parent by passing that responsibility on to Andrew.

The thing is, he probably didn't realise I was holding back and being complicit because of the inner turmoil and confusion I had when dealing with conflict. He didn't know the mess that was happening inside my mind and the paralysis I felt when he spoke with such conviction and authority. As I had done so many times in so many different circumstances, whether with teacher, work colleague, boss or parent, I froze and became blank with fear of speaking out. I know how ridiculous this might sound, but I know that to many reading this, it sounds familiar. I also know that all of the people in my life who have been the ones whom these circumstances and stories relate to, may have an entirely different perspective of the same situation. You see, behind the smokescreen of the chaos inside, is a mask of confidence, an easy-going attitude and often agreement, perhaps sometimes some discussion around options, but usually agreement. This is what makes the situation bearable and it allowed me to escape the confrontation, and the traumatising discovery of my processes, from being seen.

I realise now that I had been holding onto tons of resentment and anger. It was all suppressed, and the place it was being held in my body, was my liver, hence the anaemia. I had been living a life of agreeable confidence, outwardly showing absolute competence and confidence in every area of my life and tucking feelings of resentment away.

Continuing to live like this would lead to sudden and uncontrollable mini breakdowns. These breakdowns would always occur in safe places. It reminds me of my daughter and her 'safe tantrums'. She hated walking around shopping centres and would just stop and either stand still, refusing to walk any further, or throw herself down in a display of iron-willed authority and defiance. But there was always a careful way in which she 'fell' down, and it never resulted in any pain or injury. And so with my own mini breakdowns, they were often expressed in massive outbursts of uncontrollable sobbing and collapsing in emotional pain - this was usually done when I was out on a run, or safely in the shower with no one home, or very often in the car behind sunglasses and blaring radio.

The more unhappy I became, the more I wanted to escape from the pain that being in my relationship was causing me, and inadvertently also my husband, even though he wasn't privy to the details behind the scenes. I remember one time I was talking to my daughter in my room and needed to have a quick shower, so we continued the conversation with her sitting on the bed and me in the ensuite shower. As I finished, I stepped onto the bathmat, grabbed my towel, face planted aggressively into it and began drying myself very roughly and heavily. I don't remember when I began doing this, but my daughter was taken back, asking me why I was being so aggressive towards myself. I hadn't seen it, but it was there, self-aggression. I was literally punishing myself in small ways every single day because I was carrying around a huge load of repressed anger and confusion.

Another time I recall was after dinner one night. I was finishing cleaning up in the kitchen and Andrew called me to sit and watch the movie with him and the boys. I kept fussing and saying I was coming soon, and eventually I sat down next to him on the couch. At one stage he looked at me, and noticed I was clenching my fists tightly and asked why I was doing that. I remember that I wasn't even taking in the movie, I had been sitting there feeling so tightly wound up with emotions that the world around me was inconsequential, I was in my own little world of pain, feeling sad, anxious and definitely not present in the moment.

I could never show or talk about my outbursts to my husband because I didn't know how to talk about what was behind them. I was living a secret, a lie, a shameful and deceitful mess of confusion that just kept growing, because the small outbursts I allowed myself were not enough to balance anything out.

TEN

SAMEHA AND MARIANNE

Sameha and Marianne were two very important people who came into my life in the early 2000s. Sameha became my monthly massage therapist, after being introduced to her by Andrew. She would come to our home and spoil us with her magic touch. I didn't realise she was very connected to spirit, especially since this was before any of my personal growth into spirituality.

When I was pregnant with my last baby Daniel, she invited me to her home to indulge me in a pregnancy massage. I was around 11 weeks and had only just found out the sex of the baby a few days prior. Andrew and I decided not to tell anyone yet though, and we also chose the name Daniel for our brewing bundle.

I was completely taken by surprise when Sameha began asking me questions as she was performing some healing Reiki on me.

First, she asked if I knew the sex of the baby, to which I replied no, since I'm very good at keeping secrets. After a few moments she told me that 'they' said it's a boy, definitely a boy. Okay, I thought, this is a little weird, but interesting. Then she asked if we had thought of names. Again, I replied that no we hadn't. Again, she told me that 'they' were telling her that his name would be Daniel. It didn't stop there. The next thing she told me was that I was going to have a very quick birth, since he was in a hurry to be here. Well my first birth was via a planned Caesarean section, and the two subsequent births weren't exactly quick, around eight hours (plus) of labour each.

Fast forward to the birth of Daniel and it was only two hours from the time my waters broke until my baby boy was in my arms. I found Sameha's gift to be incredible, she was so connected and psychic. In fact, I didn't let her in on how accurate she had been until quite some time after Daniel was born. She wasn't surprised but was interested in why I hadn't told her sooner, or even at the time. I explained that I was probably too shocked to be hearing the details of a conversation that was private, being told back to me. Oh, and the biggest synchronicity of all, as if there needs to be more, is that Daniel was born on Sameha's birthday, November 25, a Sagittarius. So now we had two fire signs – Emily a Leo, Daniel a Sagittarius – and two water signs – both Angela and Ryan are Cancer, born two days apart. Add that to my Earth sign of Taurus and Andrew's Pisces, and we have a pretty interesting mix.

Sometime in the next couple of years Sameha was massaging me and asked, "What are you running away from?"

It took me by surprise, and I replied that I was running because it was fun and I loved triathlon and competing.

She wasn't buying this at all and reminded me a few times that she believed I was running away from something in my life I didn't want to face.

How right she was, but it would take me much longer to actually hear those words properly and for them to really resonate. It seems very ironic that now Sameha is a regular attendee of my meditation classes and loves the potent healing energy that I emit.

Around this time, I was at a point that I admitted I probably needed some counselling. I kept myself so busy with my training schedule that it filled my life when I wasn't being a mother and wife, so my mental health took a back seat in my awareness, acknowledgment and attention to it. It was in the year prior to our business collapsing so I wasn't coping well some days. Sameha recommended someone she had received a great review from, by a family member.

I called Marianne, who I found out was a clinical psychologist and kinesiologist, with a very holistic approach utilising alternative methods in her sessions. I found her approach to be so well rounded that I still have sessions with her when I feel the need.

When she tapped into the subconscious voice inside of me in my initial session, I broke down into sobs. I didn't believe I had a connection to my soul anymore and she led me back to believing in myself, connecting to my intuition and revealing so much more than I ever knew about the destructive inner programs I held onto. I had learned prior to this that the order in which you are born into a family affects your personality traits, and even deep seeded fears and emotions that consistently show up in your life.

Being the third of four children, and my arrival meaning Mum had three very young children, a newborn, a two-year-old and a (just) three-year-old. Now while I haven't spoken in depth with Mum about her emotional health at that time, I can imagine it would have been pretty hectic physically as well as draining mentally and emotionally.

Dad was a true provider so was up with the sparrows and home in time for dinner and then very early to bed, therefore Mum had the sole parent duties all day every day. We only ever got a little play time with Dad, and my most vivid memories of very early years were of when he took us to bed on his shoulders and let us bounce around on the mattress before settling in. The other one was of Friday nights when he would bring small white paper bags filled with lollies for each of us. My favourites were the chocolate bullets, the chocolate stars, the freckles and the cobbers which were chewy caramel in chocolate.

From the kinesiology – which I feel is in the realm of regression therapy, since in those sessions I have visited places from my life that I had not remembered at all, simply by tapping into my subconscious and all it holds – I had the opportunity to feel into how my earliest weeks, months and years have shaped me. It was revealed that I picked up on Mum's emotions, and perhaps on one or maybe more occasions, I felt the desperate need to be quiet, so as not to upset an already tired, perhaps exhausted mother. I know all mothers will relate to the overwhelming exhaustion and emotional fatigue at times with little ones. Mum has never mentioned post-natal depression and I don't remember any evidence of it, so this memory is purely for my own inquiry as to early incidents which had a very real effect on my beliefs.

As I continued down the path of my kinesiology/counselling sessions, I found that memories would come back in waves. For many years I could recollect almost no childhood memories, although I didn't realise this until I really began listening. Listening when my sister would recall stories from our childhood, names and places and events that I could definitely relate to, like knowing who she was talking about, where we were living etc, but could not for the life of me, find in my memories. My mind had blocked so many memories and I wanted to know why. Why did I have armour around my memories, or my heart? What was I afraid of?

This recognition of hidden and elusive memories was ignited only after spending a few years unlocking other parts of me through kinesiology, meditation, seeking out books and podcasts and YouTube channels to answer burning questions that I didn't even know I had. I simply followed my insatiable thirst for knowledge and answers.

After a while, my desire for answers became insignificant, I now had a burning need for deep knowing and connection to God, or source or the Universe. I didn't care anymore about giving this massive force a name, I let go of my religious beliefs of adhering to one aspect of what this universe has to offer. I wanted to feel like my soul had purpose, I wanted to feel held by what I knew existed inside my very being, beyond the physical body I was in and beyond any restrictions that any religion has placed upon me. I yearned for the fleeting feelings of my childhood, lost in prayer during Sunday Mass, when I felt at peace, on a level that had me in raptures of love like I had never felt before.

Now I was thrashing and forging a path in my psyche that required diligent focus and repetition. The questions were still there, they had been my trigger point leading to the quest for answers, leading to the forming of questions, leading to the divinely timed synchronicities. Synchronicities such as walking into a Vinnie's store (St Vincent de Paul Society) after a chiropractor appointment.

I remember thinking, *I wonder if they would have some spiritual books that would be helpful for me?* At that time, I had been listening to, no, I was addicted to and spent every minute I could, listening to Abraham Hicks, a channeled voice of the collective consciousness who spoke into my very soul, or so it seemed. I had already purchased a couple of their books, so I knew what I was looking for. I walked into the store and went straight to the bookshelves.

The heavens opened and rained down upon me a collection of near new books from spiritual authors I had and hadn't heard of. The Seth books, another channeled series and there were about five of these. Robin Sharma and Paolo Coelho, both masters at storytelling, and several more of the Abraham books. They were all there, in this tiny and out of the way secondhand store in the outlying suburbs of Sydney. I purchased and devoured these books. They spoke to me and were perfect for what else was happening in my life.

At a time where I was truly searching for meaning, answers and guidance, this was not only perfect, but shouted loudly to me that my yearning had been heard. When I break down what that yearning looked like, it wasn't a place of desperation or lack that it was coming from. It was a place of truly desiring more of the same, only more and more applicable to exactly what I needed to know to grow more into my soul. I had a true desire to be more, even though I didn't know what that even meant, but I knew that by listening to my intuition it would lead me somewhere I was meant to be.

In my life I was, once again, learning to be small. Like when I was a child. I desperately wanted to be seen and heard but when opportunities arose, I felt like I had nothing of value to offer. I was now at a stage in my life where the challenge was real, and I was losing myself on one level, while focusing wholeheartedly on another aspect that kept me fulfilled physically and mentally. That is, I was training regularly, doing lots of races and travelling to compete which also included family involvement and weekends away. I felt so healthy, fit and fulfilled. Yet I was avoiding a situation around me that was unfolding and needed attention. In a word. I felt. POWERLESS.

I've never handled confrontation well. In fact, I hate it. I melt down and can't think straight. I feel overwhelmed, belittled, outsmarted and targeted. All rationality seems to abandon me as I grow smaller into submission. That makes it difficult for the other person since they don't know my inner turmoil and often get frustrated at my avoidance and seeming flippancy in these moments. It's something I'm constantly working on, and I believe I'm getting much better at. I realise this is something I desire, and require, to wrestle to the ground and talk to in a primal and deep way while we are in a locked grip. I want us to be bound together to get to the bottom of this, once and for all, with no escape route into avoidance. I want this voice to speak sincerely to me, it's an armour that I've placed around my heart and soul for protection from – well, that's what I want to figure out.

As I have begun wrestling with this, I chose to allow my trusted confidante Marianne to guide me, through my own body, into some of the deeply held belief structures this behaviour has stemmed from. And here are some of the beliefs I had been holding onto:

- If I get my own needs met, others are disadvantaged.
- Others drain me of my energy, I also drain others of their energy.
- There is no way out. I'm stuck.
- My needs are secondary.
- I judge my needs.
- In order to keep the peace, I have to move away from my own truth and allow others to win.
- I must give all I have to the person/people closest to me in order to be loved.
- It's hard, almost impossible to say NO.

So, I'll try now to paraphrase these deeply embedded, DNA level beliefs that I have carried around with me for who knows how long, to give an insight into this life that I never dreamed I would be living.

To pre-empt the following words, it's important to note that much inner work including self-healing, meditation, rituals, courses, holidays and spiritual adventures, dialogue with my trusted mentor and a staunch vow to become the very best version of who I am, has all been melded into this synopsis.

I couldn't decide on anything I wanted to be or do when I was approaching completing high school. The facts I had to work with included that I had a serious boyfriend, my first, and he was stable financially and emotionally, lots of fun to be around and loved me to the very core. I had no big plans for my life other than knowing I would be a mother, that was a certainty.

But it was brought to the test when I was only 15 years old. That's when I decided to use food as my source of control. It felt so good to be in control of my weight, it just melted off me when I starved myself. It was so easy, just get used to eating hardly anything and then I would look good and people would notice me. I wasn't sure why I craved to be noticed because I didn't have anything to prove. I gave no thought to any future issues of lack of nutrients, it just really suited me to feel good in my body and to finally fit into my sister's clothes.

Of course, it drove my mother crazy, with no knowledge or publicity around eating disorders she felt helpless in her attempts to encourage me to eat, as I pushed food around my plate. I recall lying on the floor in the lounge room one evening, watching television and I looked down at my legs. The little fat that was on my thighs was annoying me because it made me think that I needed to lose it. I would need to jog around the football field more and eat less. These were the thoughts that consistently played in my mind, always around my weight and my food intake. Food really was my enemy, and it was all consuming. If I wasn't eating, I felt good. If I did eat I would be thinking of how I could burn those calories off, and I was constantly lying about what and how much I ate to my mum.

One day changed that story abruptly. It was a school day and before I walked out the door, Mum asked if I needed any sanitary supplies. She thought that surely, I must since she didn't remember buying any for me in recent months. I thought about what I would say in reply since I had silently been quite worried, but I thought I should tell the truth – so I said, "Mum, I haven't had my period for nine months now."

I guess my body fat was so low that my body didn't want to waste energy on the reproductive system generating a possible new human to nourish. When I got home from school that afternoon, Mum had made a doctor's appointment to get to the bottom of this. I was happy to go since I was concerned just as much as Mum.

As I walked into the male doctor's office, he asked me to go and pee into a small cup, which I did. After a few minutes he told me that I definitely wasn't pregnant. Well I could have told him that! I was so embarrassed, had this doctor thought that I was having sex? Oh my God!! How totally humiliating for me! My religious upbringing and beliefs surrounding sex resulted in me subconsciously and consciously holding a lot of shame around sex, seeing it as shameful, especially if you get pregnant as a teenager.

He went on to ask me about my eating habits, and I was truthful, telling him I had been dieting but not offering much more. His next words altered my life direction. He told me that I had a choice: either I begin eating three healthy meals a day, or I might be at a very high risk of never being able to have children.

Okay, I let that sink in for a minute. But I didn't even need a minute. I already knew that the diet days were over, I would listen to his recommendation and begin eating healthy, which I did that very day. In fact, I was so relieved to be told that I had to eat normally again that I didn't even need reminding by Mum. This makes sense because I had been out of control, but I didn't want to be seen as failing at being skinny, I now had a legitimate reason to turn the all-consuming behaviour around. I didn't go into overdrive and eat everything in sight since I wasn't bulimic, but I made sure I ate a diet rich in nutrients, just like I always had been encouraged to anyway.

Since then I have always been very aware of empty calories in my diet and choose not to include them very often. The main offenders like chocolate, chips, biscuits, alcohol and all processed food. Moderation was and is my key, as is listening to my body's cravings.

Some days I'll eat mostly fruit simply because my body is starving for it, or so it seems. The point is, I listen to it, and when I do, there are simply no cravings for the damaging nutrient-free and chemically laden, fat and processed-sugar dense foods that are constantly thrown at us via manipulative advertising and easy access and availability.

The story obviously has the happy ending of four beautiful and healthy children being born into this world through my body. Diagnosis of eating disorders usually boils down to taking back control. That certainly rings true for me. But just as I had taken control in starving my body, I also took back control to nurture my body. I feel very blessed to have had such a strong connection to unborn children that I turned my situation around.

When I went into past life and current life regression in my sessions using methods of kinesiology to take me back to certain time frames in my life my childhood played a significant part in determining my long-held beliefs. One such session went like this. After determining where I needed to visit on my life's timeline, I was taken back to being a very young baby. So, there I was as an infant, voicing my needs for milk, affection or comfort through crying. And in that one (or more) instance, I was met with a response which went something like this: I was needy and I vocalised this, and something bad or very distressing happened either to me or to the person I am totally dependent on for life. It could have been that I was waiting longer than usual and thought I had been abandoned, or it could have been that Mum was distressed and overwhelmed and I picked up on this, it could have been a number of scenarios. And bang... a belief was formed in that instant. The belief that told me that if I was needy or even vocal in displaying my needs – and later my opinions – something bad might happen. The accompanying belief was that I needed to read the other person to know what it was that would make them happy (people pleasing). Simple as that.

This belief then grew tentacles and hooks in my subconscious, and then as I grew older, every event in my life where I 'caused' an angry or frustrated reaction in someone else made me feel frozen in fear. And this made total sense to me. It described perfectly how I felt, and still sometimes feel, when in confrontational situations, or where my input and decision is required.

My husband used to get really frustrated with me in restaurants because of how long it took for me to decide what I wanted to eat. It was ridiculous behaviour and I still find it difficult making those decisions, but I know now, that I was acutely aware of our financial situation throughout our marriage, and wanted to order something well within the budget, but I didn't actually verbalise this. I ordered something other than what I would have if I hadn't seen the prices. Often it made me angry afterwards because he would then order an expensive dish as if we had all the money in the world – this was the underlying language in my mind. This is still one that springs up at times, but it's getting better, and my money language improved enormously once I left my marriage.

In 2008 one of my personal training clients recommended I contact a spiritual kinesiologist who ran meditation classes, since during our conversations I'd told her about the methods Marianne used and how intrigued I was with learning more about spirituality. I contacted this woman and had some sessions with her, and then went on to participate in her group meditations each Tuesday evening. She had me mesmerised with her channeling and connection to spirit both in private sessions and in group meditations.

So profound was the energy and discussion of everyone in the room, all of whom were deeply spiritually aware and many quite psychic, our group transformed into what was known as the Ascension Group. Our meditations weren't structured since being unplanned and in the moment allowed for a constant connection to the energy within the room. I absolutely loved those weekly sessions and counted the days from one Tuesday 'til the next, I was a sponge for all that energetic healing energy and the channeled messages from spirit. I was shifting and growing from these experiences and allowing myself to open up to something I had been conditioned to stay away from in accordance with the Catholic Church. But what I was receiving was often euphoric and it made me feel so comforted and at home in myself.

One day I walked into the centre and there were only a few people there as we were setting up the room. There was the most beautiful fragrance enveloping the room, not overpowering but definitely an incense-like aroma unlike anything I had ever smelled.

I commented to the owner of the centre, who had been working there all day, how I loved the incense she was burning. She looked confused. I haven't burned incense today at all, are you sure you can smell it? It threw me since the smell was very real.

Within a few minutes she realised that what I would have been smelling would be the vibhuti of Sai Baba, an Indian Spiritual Master who has incarnated, similar to the Dalai Lama in many different generations and lifetimes. She had been on a pilgrimage only a few years prior with her sister to have an audience with him, so could vouch for his high regard with millions around the world who would flock to see him. He had a revered gift and simply being in his presence often resulted in having a spiritual experience, awakening or healing. He performed many healings in person and remotely, and would rub his hands together, materialising the vibhuti, an ash like substance, very earthy and with a unique aroma. He often instructed others to put a little on their tongue to receive or imbue its essence some other way.

Many people around the world know of it and the magic that surrounds it. It has turned up in people's mailboxes without any request or return address, it has been known to be almost depleted in the supply only to keep renewing itself. It is a mystery.

I was gifted a small portion by my teacher and have used it and given it to others many times, and there still seems to be the same amount in my container. There have been times when I was guided to place a small amount on my tongue, and then I was guided through a complete chakra cleanse which would last up to about 30 minutes.

During these sessions I surrendered to guided self-healing, where my hands created portals and moved fluently, writing sacred script in the aura around me. My energetic centres would pulsate with the potency of this ritual as I experienced great releases of stuck energy, while simultaneously an infusion of an invisible force so palpable my body would shake and quiver as it became one with me.

Transformation took place on a grand scale during these sessions, and in 2015 I was given the word 'transfiguration' to use for these processes and for my work. As happens with vital messages, they are spoken silently to me, I feel them, then if I feel the slightest resistance or doubt, they rise through me and are literally shouted out of my mouth. This was on such time, so the word Transfiguration is one I continue to use to describe my work.

After these healing experiences I would feel a purity within and would often need to rest and absorb the uplevelling I just experienced.

I was shown a picture of this happy looking man with black frizzy hair, afro style and I immediately felt his beautiful energy.

I was finding my nirvana in places and through experiences I would never have imagined.

Our teacher was also a facilitator for a Kinesiology modality, Touch for Health and since I had been touched so deeply with this practice, I enrolled to do her next course.

The time finally arrived and over several weekends our small group of students learned the techniques of muscle testing, studying the client's responses and how to relate them to the meridians needing adjusting. It was intriguing, and we practiced on each other, reciprocally giving and receiving, honing our techniques and understanding the protocols.

After receiving our certification, we practiced over the coming weekends refining and learning from each other.

Then a peculiar thing began happening. Following the guidelines of our manual, I was about to begin the movements required over a certain meridian when my arms and hands began moving involuntarily, in a beautiful flowing motion over the place of blocked energy. My whole body supported the motion, swaying into the movement and creating a flow of energy over the exact place I was meant to be working on according to the manual, but it was an involuntary movement, one that came through me, not one that I mentally prepared and executed.

As my teacher watched she commented that I was doing great. Of course, I responded that it was me, but it wasn't me, the movement was just happening, and I was allowing it. She stood back, watched and saw that it was the perfect flow and placement, and to keep going, allow the energy to flow through this Divine connection.

I was on cloud nine, I had been desiring a more tangible connection and now I was feeling it. When I began adding kinesiology in addition to my personal training sessions, I expected to be following the protocol in the manuals to the letter, thinking this would be the best and safest way to proceed.

But I soon realised that wasn't how I was meant to be using this connection I had. In no uncertain terms I was given the message to put my manuals away and focus on the person, allowing the connection to determine the process I would use, and most importantly to trust and surrender to the process. I would find myself beginning to quietly channel in the movements as my hands carried out their own energetic patterns all over the person. The more I allowed and trusted the process, the more the session flowed.

In time, I was told by Mother that the certificates were simply to satisfy my own human need for a certification, giving me permission to practice. The truth is that the most potent and effective healing modalities cannot be learned from a manual, through a course or a book, even by a mentor. The world we live in has been conditioned over the most recent centuries to abandon the most sacred healing rituals and modalities of all, discrediting them as black magic, evil, voodoo, and instead enticing the majority of the population to abandon our ancestors and choose to follow a society where if it's not backed scientifically or with studies, then it's not valid. I do believe however that all of that's on the very brink of shifting and there will be a dynamic wave flooding humanity to 'see' their Godliness within, and throw away the rulebooks that have blindsided us from our own path of truest integrity.

In light of this, I was aware of the judgment I believed I would receive, and the criticism from those who think they know everything, and this resulted in me being quite mindful of who I told about my gifts, outside the circle of my clients and the people in meditation class. I guess I held back for quite some time for fear of being ridiculed, questioned, or even worse, losing my connection and looking like a fraud, feeling like a failure.

But I had the support of my Tuesday group. I lived for those Tuesday evenings, it was like going home, in a very cosmic way. I was always transported to the most magnificent places during those sessions. My heart and soul were being fed, and they were hungry. In hindsight, the way I became so familiar with this routine is quite bizarre. Considering I had never strayed from my Catholic upbringing to include anything so mystifying as what I had experienced in this time, signified that I was indeed primed (from the self-development work I had been doing) to dive right into what had been brewing below the surface for some time.

Another aspect of this communication of my body's ability to bring this healing to others was when I began receiving answers to questions, in a yes/no nodding or shaking of my head. It began one Sunday afternoon as I was driving back from my kinesiology training. I was meeting my family at a Christening and it was in a suburb of Sydney that I was unfamiliar with. It was before the days of Google maps on our phones and I didn't have a navigation system in my car, just an old-fashioned street directory and my skills at reading those maps was dismal. I could do this.

I was driving along the motorway and as I approached an exit I thought in my mind, should I take this exit? As soon as I asked my head nodded YES very definitively. Whoa! Okay, this was new. I took the exit, and as I continued driving, I asked if this was Mother, and my head nodded firmly YES again.

I continued onto the venue of the christening by following all the prompts I was given along the way. Yes and No always being the answers to my questions of which streets to turn into. I was blown away. How could this be? And then of course, I began to think that my entire life would now change. I would simply ask questions before making decisions that I was unsure of. What a dream life I was going to have, bring it on!

Not so fast. I wasn't going to be let off the hook of being responsible for my own journey, for listening to my intuition and for feeling my way into life in it's intricacies and those moments of weighing up what felt better, rather than expecting an easy way out and becoming lazy and a living like a robot. That was exactly what I didn't want, and it would have been giving my power away completely.

However, this nodding and shaking of my head is something of a constant, and it mostly happens when I'm least expecting it. For example I could be in a client session and downloading an intense message, with interspersed conversation with the client, when a very pronounced YES via a strong nodding of my head happens, in that moment we both know this message is very intentional and that what is coming through is crucial and to really take notice. It's like a cosmic audience where there is a consensual agreement with every aspect of consciousness. It never ceases to leave me smiling and having an inner soul party. Yes, even as I write this book, the nods and the accompanying smiles that broaden and light up my entire facial expressions and often instantaneous laughing out loud are a constant.

As I continued practicing the modality of kinesiology, I was using the certificates to validate my authenticity for quite some time before 'coming clean'. Every single moment of the sessions was channeled through my body, I became more and more aligned to the movements of my body to allow and bring not only healing to others, but to the environment I worked and lived in. Often in outdoor areas when I was alone, I often moved and worked with the surrounding energy.

It took some time for me to recognise that there was no training that existed that would be responsible for teaching me what I was doing, it just didn't exist. I had learned from my own soul, from a source far greater and more powerful than any human being. I had learned how to surrender and to utilise my own body in all ways to transmute, heal and allow others to change their lives.

ELEVEN
THE NEXT UPGRADE

Working with energy and acknowledging my healing abilities had become more ingrained into me as the months went by. It was as if I had grown into my shoes and clothes properly, the sort of feeling where everything seems so normal and so right that life before my gifts were revealed seemed so long ago. Yet I may have underestimated how the new branches of these gifts would unfold.

One day in 2010 something rather interesting happened. As I was going about my afternoon my body turned and I stood facing a blank wall. It was a feeling I was becoming familiar with now when I was entering a phase of channelled work. A similar feeling to being out of your body and being controlled by puppet strings, but the source of the movement was not from outside of my body, it was from the inside. I want to reiterate that I never felt trapped, tricked or possessed. In fact, quite the opposite. I felt like I was stepping into a higher version of myself, a version that was aware of so much more than the physical world I was in, encompassing all aspects of me. This was the sign I was now in full connection to spirit, my highest consciousness. Almost like a light switch had been flicked and I could see so much more, only I FELT it rather than saw it, my whole body became hyper aware and sensitive in the instant of the shift.

My hands began making circular motions very close to the wall, the intensity picked up and it became quite a workout over the next hour or so, it could have been much more or much less. All concept of time was lost as I entered into these states of other worldly consciousness. The circular patterns grew and then they were reversed, persisting until I had covered all four walls of the room. Mixed in with the circular motions, I was then making vertical and horizontal motions over the entire room, then the floor, then the ceiling. It was like a frenzy and my head was spinning a little too, with the intensity as well as the almost out of body experience I was having.

I repeated this process over every square inch of that four-bedroom home over the next few weeks. I remember clearing stale and stagnant energies that were projecting in certain areas of the home as well, and the dining room was where several such portals needing a massive shake up. That's where things went next level again.

This time I began slowly twirling, gaining a little momentum, then a little more, then more, more, more until I thought I was going to be flying. Since I had agreed to enter this greater aspect of myself there was no turning back when the going got tough. I can't begin to tell you how fast I was spinning around, it's fortunate that I have a good sense of balance and along this journey I learned to focus my gaze on one place as a ballerina would do when pirouetting.

Finally, I would begin slowing down, down, down and the wondrous realisation occurred that I wasn't in the least bit dizzy. Grateful that it had stopped, it was only a moment before I realised I was beginning to now spin in the opposite direction, repeating the process and thus completing the energetic portal which would allow light and healing energy to flow in. If I began to lose my focus and worry about falling down or throwing up it brought up a disconnect of fear, so I learned to trust – to trust implicitly. Day by day, week by week I would do every cupboard, wall, ceiling and floor, every single room until the entire house was as clear as crystal, energetically speaking. It was only then that I would begin to become crystal clear about my present situation, the choices before me.

When the environment you live in is littered with previous people's energy, seeping out of the walls and floors it can intoxicate you into a low-level state of survival rather than thriving. We had only moved into this home months before and during this time I was on a steep upward spiral in my spiritual journey, so this was an imperative step for me.

My boys were only in primary school at this stage, aged seven and ten. As I was doing this cleansing work in the house, in the deeply ingrained space I needed to be in, the boys would watch me and ask what I was doing. I told them I was communicating with the Angels and we were cleaning the energy of the house. They accepted this response, no questions asked. They politely excused themselves to ask me a question if I happened to be in the middle of a clearing cycle and were very respectful of the depth of space I was in. I was always consciously aware of my surroundings, never out of it so to speak, therefore could always either pause what I was doing, or if it was too difficult to stop I would let them know I would be finished in a few minutes, allowing the current process time to wind up.

What was interesting though, was that at no point during this entire time did my husband know I was doing this. There was no way I could explain it to him as he would probably attempt to convince me of the proof that this was either impossible or let me know his opinion based on his beliefs and knowledge – fill in the blank – anything but allowing me the space to continue in the trust I needed to hold.

The thing is, I didn't even attempt to hide my rituals from him, however when he would turn his key in the lock of our front door in the afternoon, my body would abruptly stop, the connection would be broken and I would resume my old normal as I discontinued my new normal. How bizarre, I would think. And how would I even begin to attempt explaining what I was up to? Even the boys never once mentioned it to their father, it was as if our energetic boundaries were firmly in place and there was no need to say anything to anyone else.

I knew this was no accident, there was a reason I had to enable myself, make my own decisions, take responsibility for what I allowed in and what I refused to allow in anymore. I was still attending the ascension group at this time, and I was noticing more signs in being much more psychically aware.

Incidentally, when I moved out of that home, a couple who were interested in purchasing the property asked the agent if they could sit with me for a chat, alone. I agreed, as did the real estate agent, although he seemed a little worried that I was going to reveal something negative, I imagine. As we sat they said they felt compelled to ask me about the incredible energy that was so palpable throughout the home. They described it as light, welcoming and loving, and said they felt it the moment they approached the house, and an unmistakable vibration of peace and love flowed throughout the home as they viewed it. This made sense since everything I had been doing was channeled directly through an angelic portal of energy and had eradicated and transmuted all old stale and stuck energy. I told them that I had been creating a huge energy shift using my spiritual healing and cleansing gifts, and that it had previously been quite energetically congested.

To this day I do house clearings and am directed instantly where the energy is stuck and old, as well as where old spirits are either stuck or trying to hang onto this energetic plane when they should have crossed over.

I was becoming more in tune with my connection and felt that I had begun a journey that would lead me to places that many people around me would not understand, or perhaps even support.

TWELVE
SEPARATION

The years post liquidation and losing everything of monetary value as well as having our emotional wellbeing tested to the limits took its toll on our marriage. I thought I would miss our big expensive home but surprisingly I was relieved to have moved out of it. It was a house that held no emotional attachment for me at all. Even though we had built it together as our dream home, and it being the result of building a company from the ground up into a multi million-dollar revenue machine, the truth was it was draining more than our finances.

It was at the beginning of the decline of the company, in 2005/6 that I experienced my anaemia issues which left me very drained a lot of the time. Andrew had taken an enormous blow and went on a downward spiral mentally and emotionally, so we were both preoccupied with our own struggles.

With Andrew's tenacity and brilliant business mind, along with his pride and relentless pursuit to provide well for his family, he continued building what he could from ground zero again. We navigated the four years following liquidation pretty well, but there were unresolved issues we both carried with us. We are both people who can put on very convincing masks while nursing painful inner truths. He liked to tell me everything but often it terrified me that we would never recover from this. Meanwhile we had a family to care for. The girls were becoming very independent now and they both had the drivers licences and cars, part time jobs and large social circles which saw them exploring life more than ever.

In 2008 we celebrated Emily's 18th, Angela's 21st and Andrew's 40th birthdays. Parties were Andrew's forte and he was in his element on these occasions, being bartender and socialising while also making sure everyone had a drink in their hand or food on their plate always. So as this paragraph explains, it was all happening on many fronts.

By 2009 I had succumbed to a cumulative sinking feeling at my very core. My body was physically showing the signs of shutting down at many times no matter how much I masked my deep unhappiness. I was still clueless as to the real cause of my life draining anaemia. I became very angry with myself because I felt that I should be grateful for everything I had, but what I didn't understand that that wasn't the issue. The issue was the tonne of old shadows I carried with me, they were becoming very heavy. The unspoken words that were gnawing at my insides, the confusion of feeling ungrateful or petty when trying to explain myself yet not knowing how to articulate the pain I carried, feeling less and less present in my marriage to the point of numbness, mind and body.

When you're carrying all of this and feel the shame it brings, the only option is to pull out the happy mask each day, then safely go back to breaking down in private, usually when I was in the shower, or when I went out for a run and just cried the whole way as I pounded out what little energy I could muster. I wasn't loving to myself and was becoming aggressive in my personal behaviours, like ploughing my face into my towel after showering and aggressively applying moisturiser and brushing my hair. My self worth was bottoming out, I was in a constant state of anxiety and it was exhausting. I was punishing myself because I didn't want to face what I knew was coming. Its' very difficult to write about this time since it was also one of the happiest times we shared. It's a true paradox.

Our boys were at a beautiful stage in their lives, both in primary school and growing into their own unique characters and personalities.

We had a few little rituals that we all loved. Friday night was movie night. We would walk to Video Ezy and rent seven movies for $10 to get us through the week, spending up to an hour carefully selecting our individual quota. We watched a movie together after enjoying a dinner of pizza or burgers. There was also bedtime stories. I loved using different voices for each character in the books I read, while Andrew often told his own concocted stories and named this series "The adventures of RyDan". I loved this character, the combined essence of both Ryan and Daniel which made it equally special for them both. The boys would eagerly await the adventures that RyDan got up to as Andrew carefully curated daring feats, near escapes and wild adventures.

Another ritual we had was a morning cup of tea. Andrew and I woke before the boys most mornings and would quietly go to the kitchen and make tea, then take it outside and sit on the verandah to take in the early moments of the day, chatting quietly so we didn't wake the boys.

Life has so many facets and I would have given anything to keep our family together. But when I faced the reality, my inner self was dying and no matter what I did to retrieve her, she wouldn't budge back into life while still being married to Andrew, or as he pointed out to me, maybe it was just that I didn't want to be married at all. Whatever it was, I had to make the toughest decision of my life and tell him I had spent everything I had, on every level, and I was so drained I had nothing left to give.

I remember the day well that we initiated our separation. We woke on a Sunday morning and when we rolled to each other I realised my tank was empty. He asked me what was wrong, and I replied, "I don't think I have anything left to give."

He asked me if I thought that I didn't, or if I actually didn't have anything left. It was the most excruciating moment of my life as I sat on that question. I couldn't lie any more. I told him I had nothing left to give. He took me in his arms and we just laid there, softly crying as we comforted each other.

After some time, we got out of bed, the boys were up and playing so we made them breakfast, then they went off to play again as we sat down to our own breakfast.

I'll always remember the emotional breakdown we had at the table that morning. We sobbed, grieving the loss so deeply of our relationship, our union, holding each other as we did so. He told me to not feel bad because it wasn't fair on him either to stay in a marriage where he wasn't loved and desired unconditionally. I'm grateful for those words.

He knew I had spent a great deal of time and energy on my personal growth and overcoming my inner demons over the past eighteen months. We had been to marriage counselling for several sessions with two different counsellors, we had tried to re-capture the essence that seemed to have been depleted.

We spent the day together, talking, crying, holding and comforting each other on this sad day. We held hands as we walked around the park, discussing the logistics of moving forward with separating, how it would work with the boys and who would move out of the house. We made some big decisions on that day which gave us a solid foundation for moving forward, apart but still connected deeply and as co-parents to the most important aspect of the future – our boys.

I think we did it well. It hasn't been easy at times and since we both have love and respect for each other, it's been difficult watching each other move on with seeing other people. But as time passes it has become much easier to accept and acknowledge each other's role in our lives as one that we have both grown and evolved into better people. He stood by me each day of our marriage with pride and encouragement in every endeavour I undertook, just as I had loved and supported him, his decisions and respected his business acumen, his nurturing personality and charisma with everyone he came into contact with. His desire to live a joyful life filled with adventure, desire and a constant yearning to become a better version of himself still inspires me.

I have many incredibly romantic memories of our relationship; it really was a passionate love affair that we had. I have learned that when you're with someone for a long time it's the little gestures of intimacy that leave an indelible imprint on your heart.

One such example was when I was experiencing terrible fatigue with anaemia and my eyes would get so sore at night that I couldn't keep them open to read my book in bed. I asked Andrew if he would read to me, I didn't mind if it wasn't my book, so he began reading to me while I lay falling asleep. Call me crazy but I found that to be one of the most intimate times and it stays firmly in my memories. It has taken me a very long time to overcome the idea of failing at relationships. I can't compare myself to anyone else or the ideals of society, and when I chose to embrace everything I gained in my marriage, I understood that I wasn't a failure. I was being true to myself and in doing so, opening up a world of opportunity for us both. As Andrew said, it wasn't fair for me to feel unhappy and guilty, and it also wasn't fair for him to be in a marriage where he wasn't loved and desired just as much as he loved and desired me.

After breakfast on the Sunday, we went for a walk around the nearby oval, around our neighbourhood, holding hands all the way and talking about the way forward from here. I don't know how long we were out walking but we just wanted to keep going, it was therapeutic for us. We were going away in a couple of weeks for a holiday to our favourite destination, Diamond Beach, just a few hours' drive north and we would tell the boys our decision there. That day was equal in the intensity to the morning a few weeks prior. The pain that we all felt was palpable. Everyone cried, of course, the boys had no idea and couldn't believe it. They were only 11 and eight years old and I felt like the worst person in the world doing this to them. We never ever went to that place again; the boys have both said that it holds so much pain they couldn't bear to go back.

In the weeks following, he searched for a suitable place to rent and secured something quite close by. The move went smoothly and as much as I wanted to help settle him in by unpacking at least the kitchen, he told me no. He had to do this by himself, we had to cut some cords and move on from each other in the little ways too. It was so lonely without him, and more so when the boys weren't with me.

Time went by and we found a rhythm with the new arrangements. Then something quite unexpected happened. I began feeling strong emotions for him, like I hadn't felt for a long time. I longed for intimacy with him like we used to have and tried to work out in my own head what was going on, but the emotions wouldn't recede. It wasn't long before we began being intimate again, more passionately than ever, it was like we had rewound the clock 15 years while also having all of those 15 years of experience knowing each other inside and out. It was like a rebirth for our relationship, we were seeing each other more, and we would explore this connection and become lost in each other. It began to look like we were headed for a reunion and we even began talking about moving back together. I didn't know what had happened, but it made me so happy.

Before making any decisions, he told me we should hold off on any more intimacy for a month, and then see if we both still felt the same. I was sure that I would, and so we stuck to that agreement. After that month, we saw each other again, and I was devastated to feel empty again. It was like whatever we had rekindled had completely disappeared. I tried desperately to feel into what I had felt just a month before, but my heart just wouldn't or couldn't go there again, I couldn't find it. We were both so saddened. I know that I was distressed at what was happening, but I also knew I could never ever pretend again, especially not with him.

We agreed that counselling might be a good idea, and over the following several weeks we turned up to our appointments, both being honest about our feelings. Counselling hadn't been helpful for me in the past, and this time was no different. I felt misunderstood, even though both the counsellor and my husband were doing their best to understand my feeble attempts to explain my deep pain and anguish. I told him I could no longer do this, nothing was shifting and if anything, I was feeling certain that I had made the right decision for me, for us, to separate. He had desperately wanted to connect with the "me" who had shown up in those few weeks when we found a place full of love, and I just as desperately wanted to be able to find that place again, but I couldn't.

For months after separating, I continued to work casually at the health club, for the sole reason that I had little confidence in knowing how I would support myself and the boys financially now that I was a single parent. Even though I had done this successfully before, I still felt attached to the security of a job that would require regular contact with Andrew. I knew it was time for me to move on, and I was about to be given a shove in no uncertain terms.

We both agreed it was hampering our efforts to move on while this situation continued, but I still clung to a few shifts a week, until something strange began happening. As I was working, I would experience extreme pressure in my head, like a vice was tightening. Since I don't suffer from headaches, I didn't know what this was, but then when

I left the building, the pressure immediately ceased. Interesting. Then it happened again and again, until I really listened to the message I was receiving, to stay away, to build my life outside of what I had become accustomed to. I finally made the decision to leave completely, it was so hard, cutting the final tie to 'us'.

THIRTEEN

THE INNOCENCE OF SPIRIT IN CHILDREN

As our lives continued to unfold as co-parents, doing the best we could to give the boys and ourselves the best home life possible under the circumstances that divorce brings, things sometimes popped up when we relied on each other's support. One morning I received a call from Andrew telling me that Daniel wasn't well, and could he bring him over to my house while he goes to work.

Shortly after, the three of them arrived to drop Daniel off. He was only seven years old and had been ill through the night with a gastric bug. He hadn't been able to keep anything down, or in for hours. Even water would come right back up, so I placed him on my lounge to rest and keep an eye on him, intending on taking him to the doctor. I offered him a few sips of water and sure enough, it came back up within seconds. I intended to take him to the doctor but was really feeling like I needed to do some healing work on him.

As I stood over him, channeling through a Divine energy through my vocal sounding and movement through his auric fields, he slept soundly and heavily. He awoke a couple of hours later from his slumber. I gave him some water to sip. He kept it down. Soon after I gave him a small amount of food and he kept it down as well. Now you may be thinking this was simply the course of the bug, and I understand that because I did too. And the next few days went by uneventfully with him having fully recovered since the moment he woke up.

Out of the blue, he began to tell me that he hadn't yet told me about what he felt and saw when I was doing my healing work around him on that day. I listened curiously as he began to tell me how, as soon as I began, he saw a face appear in front of him, a large white face, he wasn't scared, it was just there. Then the face began to separate into many, many faces surrounding him, all white. Then they seemed to elevate a little more, and in a swooping cyclonic rush, they disappeared into his stomach, whooshed right up through his body and out of the crown of his head. In that moment he felt calm, and immediately went into a deep sleep. I absolutely love that he was able to relate that to me, with such innocence and detail, at the tender age of seven. And I truly believe that had he not witnessed my behaviour in the previous months, working with the angelic realm, always letting him know what I was doing all those days when I was energetically clearing our home, that he would not have been to articulate or even communicate what he experienced.

He also came to me another time after this incident and excitedly told me he had a vision of little fat white angels with arrows floating in the air. Okay, I said, they're probably cherubs. Oh, okay, but then there was another bunch of red ones, and these ones weren't good, they were bad. They had funny forks in their hands, and they were throwing them at the good ones above. I listened, and he seemed to have finished the story, so I tried to say that maybe the bad ones really were good, maybe he misunderstood. Silly me, why would I interrupt my boy's story like that! Trying to change his vision? But he wasn't finished and corrected me saying they were definitely evil. As the fork throwing continued and the cherubs began throwing their arrows back at the devils, he noticed something strange was happening. As soon as a fork hit one of the cherubs, it would immediately turn into an arrow and would fire directly back at the little devil, at which point it morphed from devil to cherub! It appeared that the negative energy, when fired into and received by pure energy, was alchemised and deflected back, thereby using the force of low level frequency to feed the intensity of the higher vibrational frequency and injecting it into the source from whence it originated!

He then went on to say that after he saw all that unfold, he saw himself floating as a large white energy, above his physical body. Then this large white version of him began floating back down towards him, he felt a jolt, and then a definite reconnection back to his current reality. I've obviously used descriptive words he would not have used in the re-telling, however he is standing right beside me as I write this, as a 16-year-old, recalling the story like it was yesterday. I loved the message this vision had brought to my boy, what a beautiful and raw treat for me to receive. And then he was off again, back to playing now that he had told me about it.

Over the years he has described my auric field to me, relayed messages to me from Mother – my spiritual companion – and helped me clear many, many blockages when I ask him. He seems to know just what to do. Like the many times when I was driving – the usual place for 'things' to happen – and asked him to help relieve some of the pressure at the side of my head. He knew exactly what to do since he had seen me do it many times before. It always begins with a heaviness in my head, then it feels like pressure is building up and I'm guided to begin pulling energy out of my ears, like a long string, meters and meters of it. As this happens the relief I feel is so incredible but if I stop before the process is complete it builds up again.

On the occasions I was driving when this happened, I asked Daniel to do it for me since I needed to focus on the road. I'm sure this is a huge cosmic joke, teaching me how to teach my boys the intricacies of working with this energy, and having fun doing so. Daniel begins pulling a thread from my ear and I groan with relief. He describes it as murky brown in colour and just a long slimy thread of energy. It must represent a buildup of old material I no longer require which has just been blocking me from receiving more of what I do desire. I love how it's always about creating space for the new and unexplored, getting rid of the old and worn out ideas and imprinted behaviours we have learned.

By this time my eldest son Ryan was 12 or 13, my boys are three and a half years apart. He was really embracing a beautiful spiritual awareness and harnessing a deep psychic connection. He often described visions he had and the more he allowed his connection, the more vivid his visions became. When he described seeing through his third eye I was always listening intently, on the edge of my seat with awe and wonder at his gift. He would relay messages from Mother to me via these visions. It was beyond words, to witness something so precious yet underdeveloped in so many of our children. It's not to embarrass him but to allow others to know what is possible when the freedom of spirit allows you to open up to receiving and utilising your innate gifts.

As a young high school student, he formed a small group of close friends. They knew each other from primary school but only now were they connecting on a deeper level of friendship. Just the three of them. I'm so proud that now they are all either studying or working, they still remain close friends, and have added to their circle. Definitely a lifetime bond and all truly wonderful young men. So, in those early years these three young men would often sit under a tree during recess and lunch and talk. Ryan was open in his conversation about his third eye visions and the boys wanted in. They wanted to know how to do this, and so they began tuning in via closing their eyes, being still and quiet, and just receiving what came. They would sit for several minutes like this, and then they would all discuss their visions, if they had any. They all had visions and messages, and although I'm not sure how long this lasted, I'm so proud of them all for tuning into their spirituality at this impressionable age.

My father passed away in 2010 and I would sometimes talk to the boys about him, and his decline into Alzheimer's during the last nine years of his life. In Dad's final days, the nursing home called Mum to say he had experienced a turn. Months before, we had all agreed to not give Dad life support or lifesaving treatment should anything like this happen. Who would want to prolong death when life was nothing short of being cared for 24/7 and in a declined mental and physical state? We knew it was what he would have wanted.

So, my brothers and sister and I, along with Mum stayed with Dad almost around the clock for those four days until he passed. Somewhere during that time, I remember Dad putting his hand to his head like he was in pain. He was unresponsive and unconscious, but the pain was bringing him back. The nurses discovered that his oxygen tank was empty, but he had still been breathing through a mask attached to the tank. I can't even begin to imagine the pain he must have been in. It was quickly rectified but the headache was obviously lingering. I thought that massaging Dad's temples would relieve him, so I stood behind him at the end of his bed and rubbed his head. Then bam, his hand flew up and landed smack on top of mine, grabbed it and directed it to the centre of his forehead, he patted my hand again, and then I began massaging exactly where the pain was. He became much more settled. This was the most communication Dad had expressed in a long time and it was so very meaningful for me.

As I was sitting with Ryan one evening before he went to sleep, I was re-telling this story, getting him to role play with me and I played Dad in that scene. As I put my hand on top of his, just like Dad had done with me, Ryan jolted a little and began connecting to Dad's spirit, and then began speaking to me as Dad. He was channeling, and he was in complete allowance and trust of the situation. I was wondering if it was truly happening and enjoying the little chat with Dad. He was telling me how proud he was that I was doing the work I was meant to do; it was beautiful and emotional. And then he said something that I knew for certain that Ryan could not have known. I told Dad that I would continue to do my work as best as I could, and he replied, "That's my girl."

That's a phrase only Dad would utter to me. Then the conversation ended. Ryan was back to himself and we talked about what just happened. I thanked him for allowing Dad to talk through him, and he said that it felt so strange that he thought he was making things up and saying them. That's what channeling can feel like, only the things you say aren't things you would even think of making up. I know from experience. He had been completely conscious and aware of what he was saying, just as I had experienced in my channeling. Tapping into another state of being, on another plane allows us to be totally present, and as time goes on it becomes fluid, the allowing becomes second nature, the connection is firmed.

Ryan was inquisitive in his spiritual development and I was just as curious to what was going on, often encouraging him to tap in to his third eye so as to allow it to open more fully and integrate his inner and outer vision. The visions he explained to me were breathtaking. He saw colours, auras and especially the energy of Mother and could relay her messages to me very clearly.

One afternoon after I had seen a few clients, I laid on the table in my healing room, feeling like I needed some recovery and allowing some time for healing on myself, which was quite common. I would lie down and feel energy being moved all around me, clearing blockages, creating and opening channels for my prana, or life force, the body's vital energy to flow freely. I loved that I was able to do this, I could experience the healings that I was offering to my clients.

As I was laying down, receiving the healing I became extremely heavy in my body, then heavier and heavier until I felt like I was made from lead. It was like I was going to fall through the floor. I noticed that my arms and legs were so heavy I couldn't lift them or even wriggle my fingers or toes. While I was okay with this because I always felt absolutely wrapped in love, I did wonder how long I would be there since I hadn't talked to the boys since I finished my sessions and that made my mind wander, wanting a time frame for this process.

Then I heard Ryan calling out my name as he was walking through the house wondering where I was. He got closer to the room I was in and I was able to mutter to him, so he heard me. I told him I was having a healing and felt like lead, so very heavy and that I couldn't move a muscle. It was difficult to even move my mouth a tiny bit. We both knew something big was going on energetically. I asked him to take a look through his third eye and to explain what he saw.

He centred himself, took a step back, and looked just above where I was lying with eyes wide, mouth open, saying, "WOW! WOOOWWWW!" Then he began to describe an extremely large angel, hovering above me, face down. We both knew it was Archangel Michael, and Ryan moved in a little and with awe in his voice he said, "Look at these feathers in his wings! They're so soft and delicate, so beautiful."

He described how the large wings were very gently, slowly rising and falling just a little. I felt so peaceful, and at this moment I felt a hot vibration in my chest and my navel. Just then Ryan told me that there were two cylinders of pulsing iridescent green energy going from the angel's heart into my high heart, and from his sacral chakra, the navel area, into mine. He continued to stay with me for a few more minutes and then left me to complete the process.

This had to be the single most incredible vision he ever shared with me, so far anyway. I always fully respected his space, even though I wanted to know every detail of every vision, but that's just my curiosity. I know it can be invasive for people to constantly ask you what you can see, what messages are you getting, what can you hear etc etc.

So often during this period of time, Ryan and I would have discussions around our visions, the energy we felt and the messages we heard and received. One constant in our conversations was Mother. She often relayed something through Ryan for me to hear, validating what I had known but perhaps doubted. One such conversation was when we were talking about my clients and how these healings were changing their lives. I wondered where my business was going, and that's when Mother said loud and clear through Ryan that the floodgates were about to open. She said I would be seeing a large number of clients; she would see to it that they found me. Well, she has never failed in delivering, and that definitely came to pass for a period of those few years until I needed a break to assess my direction, my next opportunity and challenge within the realms of my work.

FOURTEEN
HARSH LESSONS AND DISRUPTION

My spiritual group was an integral part of my life, so it was absolutely mortifying when I was kicked out of meditation. Not once, not twice, but on several occasions. Can you imagine? I mean I've never ever heard of anyone being abolished from a meditation class. But then again, these were no ordinary meditations, they were a much deeper experience that took us into places of complete surrender and propelled us deeper into our own journey.

This expulsion happened in a room of about 40 people with whom I had been regularly attending these classes each week for many, many months. As I have mentioned, I craved going to these classes each week for the peace and enlightenment they brought to me. So, it was a rude awakening to have this happen when I believed I had found my soul family with whom I would always be close to.

Several times in my life now, I have gone through times of wanting to be a part of a tribe or a group, only to become dependent on them. It's a dilemma of the times though, because in new age spirituality the gurus try to tell people to find their tribe, rather than to own their own inner guidance. In this way it's just like developing a new religion. I learned long ago it is my responsibility to know when to step away and move onto the next chapter, the next person or teacher, with whom we both will grow but not become unhealthily attached.

My healing gifts had been blossoming and I was constantly working closely with Mother, among several other ancient masters who came to guide me, including Archangel Michael and Lord Melchizedek. Sai Baba, the spirit whose essence I smelled at meditation months before, was still there too with his fun and light energy. I experienced beautiful healing experiences with all of these teachers. I've spoken about a wonderful healing experience with Archangel Michael known as the warrior Angel, the angel of protection and the most powerful of all the angels in Christianity, but a few years prior I experienced several dreams, visions and healing experiences with more angels. It began when I found a deck of Angel cards and began playing with them. I loved that I immediately felt the presence of these angels all around me. I would often play around with the cards before sleeping, doing research on which angels represented what, and they would visit me in my dreams that night.

At one time I was nudged strongly by Lord Melchizedek, known in the Bible as the King of righteousness and who had come to me in meditations and dreams regularly, and I was taken into a meditative state, or a dream state, I can't recall which one because it's difficult to differentiate the minor distinction between the two. I had been feeling his presence more and more strongly in the past week or so, but this time it was like I was being led to him. When I arrived at his grand chamber, I was asked to wait in the entrance foyer until I was beckoned to enter. I waited for some time until I was called forth into a grand crystal ballroom, an Elysian chamber which also seemed to exist in space since there seemed to be no walls or ceiling, just enormous crystals suspended above me, emanating an indulgent feeling of rapture and deep euphoria, I was standing amongst the highest degree of royalty imaginable.

As I stepped inside, I noticed others around me, then he approached me, took me into his arms and began leading me into a sacred dance. We were in a place of eviternity, the state between timelessness and temporal existence, a place where angels lie. I felt this dance was my kismet, I was dancing my destiny with the most masterful of masters. This blissful state of euphoria continued for what seemed an instant yet also an eternity. I felt his tender touch and guidance take me to places of sacred insight, as if he was sharing his universal intelligence through the flow of dance. I felt so held, so desired, so understood, so enraptured, in total trust like never before. I had misplaced my trust on so many occasions before and handed my accountability over, now it was time to step out of that pattern.

We slowed, and we stood facing each other, holding our hands together. He told me it was now time to hold myself accountable to my own greatness. I knelt before him, bowed my head, then he placed a crown upon my head saying I was to now go and show others to stand proudly and confidently through the gifts I have, the responsibility I came here with. It was time, I didn't need validation outside of myself, but I did require immovable and unshakable will to deliver this to many.

There were some incredible women and men in the group, and it was always so good to connect with them on all levels. There was definitely a level of superiority with our teacher in that she commanded attention, often in an immature way including gossip. In hindsight, since I was blinded by her loud presence and authority, as has been a pattern of mine with authoritative people during my life, her embellished persona was most assuredly a huge part of my journey. I clung to her, her words and manner, as well as taking in all that she said with wonder and respect, it was such a learning journey that continued to astonish me. This served me to a very deep level, since she had so many things right, but tested me on so many levels, which is where I fell into a free-fall to exactly where I was meant to go. To that part of myself where I was allowing others to infringe on my intuition and my desires. I just couldn't help it; I was so excited to hear every wise word and to just be in her presence. She had been what I was looking for, for I don't know how long. I wasn't about to stray from this soul haven I had found.

As I continued to attend the ascension and meditation classes I shared my unfolding story with some of the other friends I had made, all of whom were very happy and excited for me. It was such a safe space, and nothing was off limits to discuss. However, I was to discover that to embody such a powerful gift would be unsettling to our teacher. It was like she was threatened and confused at the same time. Now that I tapped into this channel, my entire being wasn't going to hide it or play down for anyone. Therefore, when my actions during meditation weren't directly in alignment with what she instructed everyone to do, I was picked on and made an example of. I wasn't deliberately ignoring her, it was just that my body – or more accurately my spirit – did not want to play with everyone else, it wanted to cause some disruption. I didn't realise at the time what a cosmic game was being played out by our own higher beings, testing us to see if we would own our own power and work this out with respect and inclusion, or revert to exclusion, victimhood and childish behaviour. The thing is that I wanted to 'behave' but the pull from my soul was much too strong and oh so beautiful. In hindsight, I know I should have walked away and I'm sure she did too, but I wasn't confident enough to do so at that point, and she obviously didn't know how to tell me she didn't want me around anymore. I had more to learn and we were in this together.

The deep intuition of my soul and connection to my body was working with the energy of the room in the highest regard of all. But she didn't see it this way, and I was made to feel embarrassed and ashamed for not conforming to her guidelines. And after all, I wasn't the one running the class, so I fell into line again. Being a good girl and downplaying my own intuition and guidance, thinking that this must have been a bad thing, that I wasn't fully connected with the higher consciousness because I was working 'against' the rules. She won. I felt ashamed and bought into the idea that I had a demonic or dark energy inside of me wanting to fight and reject the alignment of the energy she was desperately trying to bring through. The problem was that during these times I would suddenly make a move, quite involuntarily, contrary to instructions and was immediately given evil glances and the dreaded feeling that I was to be punished.

She didn't fail to punish me and told me that I was to stay away until this dark side of me could play by her rules. I was absolutely devastated. I mean, this was my weekly highlight, and it was being taken away from me. She said she couldn't do anything about it since the orders were coming from her spiritual connections. So, I obeyed, and then after four weeks I was allowed back. I was so honoured, I promised to be good. But then it happened again, and then again. I was continually being kicked out of meditation to my utter dismay and disappointment. I was told how many weeks I was to stay away each time before being assessed before the next class.

This of course, was one of my earliest experiences of being given every opportunity to own my own uniqueness and walk away in gratitude for the guidance I had been given. But since the pattern I had carried for decades was still running a strong story, I didn't believe I had the confidence or the knowing to walk away. I believed that I still needed so much more from her, so I kept going back. This was a pattern I had carried, and I would continue receiving harsh lessons that would bring me to the realisation of how deeply ingrained it was.

FIFTEEN
MACHU PICCHU 2012

This pattern continued throughout the spiritual tour to Peru in 2012. My teacher had arranged a tour to Machu Picchu, a journey for those who desired or felt called to experience the sacred energy from this holy and ancient place of wonder. There were 22 of us on the tour, and everyone was giddy with excitement during the weeks leading up to our journey. There was an even stronger force within us since it was the end of the Mayan calendar in 2012, bringing forth a new age, a rebirthing for the world as we know it. The date of 21/12/2012 represents a power number of 11 when those numbers are added together. This number is known in numerology as a gateway to the unknown, the new, the unravelling of all that we have, individually and as a collective, moving towards our intentions, dreams, wishes, goals and desires.

Everything was going smoothly as we gathered on the morning of departure at the agreed location to catch our minibus to the airport. We ended up arriving at the airport four hours before our departure. Then our flight was delayed by five hours. By the time we boarded we were over each other, or that's what it seemed like to me. We were all craving some alone time and just wanted to get there already. I don't remember much of the flight. I slept soundly the entire time. In fact, my slumber was so deep it resembled having been given a general anaesthetic. I was only shaken awake quite forcefully by my seat neighbour a few times for meals and to let someone pass to use the bathroom. I could hardly believe the first time she shook me awake to let me know I really should have something to eat.

I was sitting in the aisle seat of economy class on a full flight. As I slowly woke up, very annoyed at being woken, I realised I had a meal in front of me, I also realised the whole meal and drink service had taken place long before, and everyone else had already finished and were settling nicely, and mine was the only tray table still down with a meal on it. I've never slept so soundly and deeply, let alone on a flight. I took it as a sign of some profound inner work taking place. This happened throughout the flight, and each time I ate something or went to the bathroom I resumed my slumber, instantly blanking out into oblivion. I would like to add, I had not taken anything to help me sleep or relax, or for travel sickness, nothing at all.

Upon our arrival in Lima, those of us that were travelling alone were given random roommates. The few days we spend in Lima included day trips and tours, one of which was to the underground catacombs that have become a tourist attraction. Basilica y Convento de San Francisco de Lima is a beautiful cathedral which houses the catacombs in the underbelly of this ancient site, which was constructed between 1535 and 1649 and dedicated to St John, Apostle and Evangelist. As you can imagine, its beauty is overwhelming, stunning, and breathtaking. Works of art adorn this working monastery, true genius has touched this sacred place, and the energy is potent.

After marveling at the workmanship and dedication to this monument, we began our descent into the basement which was built to house the bodies of the wealthy residents and hierarchy of Lima who purchased the exclusive real estate to be buried and preserved in. However, as more and more wealthy Catholics died, the bodies were stacked in large concrete vats, cylindrical and very deep, where lime was poured over them and they decomposed down to the bone. Then their skeletons were separated into body parts and arranged in large square concrete containers, some were arranged in an aesthetically pleasing way for viewers to see with skulls and femurs forming a circular pattern like a flower. Other concrete containers were filled with tibias, fibulas, radius and ulnas. Walking along corridors of these body parts was eerily uncomfortable and unsettling for me, as I began feeling an intensity of emotion rising all around me, almost deafening and suffocating. It was like the spirits of the dead were calling out to be freed, released or heard. The flesh might have gone but the bones were very much alive.

As a group, and individually, some of us just held space, acknowledging the gamut of emotion that was hovering all around us, almost menacingly, doing our best to allow it to be released through our connection to the higher consciousness. The heaviness began to lift but there was still so much there when we left. I sensed anguish and despair as the primary emotions emanating from the collective 'lovely bones'.

We began forming smaller intimate groups and made our way to Cusco to acclimatise before beginning our four-day trek on the Inca Trail to our destination. It became increasingly uncomfortable to be around our group leader since her marriage was going through a tremendous strain. Her husband was on the trip and being a fabulous support to all of us, and to her in particular.

As the days went on, she began ignoring him, sleeping in her sisters room and became aggressive at times with many of us. It was obvious she was trying to hold it together and be the enlightened spiritual guide, while going through a very human struggle which was demanding her emotional strength and attention. I imagine the pressure on her to be this leader to our group was immense and dealing with an impending breakup just wasn't on the agenda.

I was found to be the disruptor during one of our meditations yet again. I was kicked out, yet again, asked to not participate in any of the group gatherings where meditation or ceremony was taking place. In other words, I was ostracised for being myself among a group of spiritual students. Since I was under the belief that there was something disruptive in me, and that this must have been a 'bad' thing, I felt that I was missing out on a huge part of the whole spiritual journey we were meant to be taking as a group.

Then we were instructed to change our roommates, even if we were happy with our current ones, since one person was matched with a disruptive insomniac roommate and couldn't get much sleep due to the constant noises and disruptions through the night. Apparently, there was rustling of bags, the taps turning off and on and the rattles of pill bottles. Some of us were discreetly told the reason, and then it was announced that everyone was going to be changing their roommates as directed by the leader of the group.

When I was allocated a new roommate, my previous one with whom I had formed a lovely friendship began ignoring me, and this went on for days. No eye contact, blatant ignorance of my presence and I couldn't understand why. It turned out that she thought I had requested to not be roomed with her and she felt abandoned after letting her guard down to me. This is an indication of the disruption of the dynamics within our group which was flowing down from the facilitator.

If I thought that the disdain I felt from the leader was all in my mind, I was about to be proven wrong. When we were all having breakfast, preparing to be picked up for a day tour to some ruins and villages, I began feeling a little off. I prepared a plate of light food and a cup of tea. As I went to eat some food, my hand wouldn't come to my mouth. It was so weird, as if there was a magnetic force in between the food and my mouth. So, I tried drinking my coca tea and the same thing happened when the cup stayed mid air and I couldn't bring it to my mouth, it was the same magnetism keeping me from ingesting anything, food or fluid. So of course, I knew this was meant to be, my body was protecting itself and I needed to fast for a period of time either to fight off a bug or to cleanse for a spiritual download.

We all boarded the bus and proceeded to the sites. I felt worse as the day progressed so decided to stay on the bus and sleep at some of the sites. By this time the situation between the group leader and her husband had escalated to a palpable and disruptive disconnection, with some people within the group having to choose sides, supporting either her or him. She should have been allocating some of the responsibilities onto her sister or close friends within the group, but her ego wouldn't let her, so she continued to try to control everything and everyone herself. When she asked why I wasn't getting off the bus to visit one of the sites I explained I wasn't feeling well. She looked at me with daggers and told me that I shouldn't have bothered coming, I should have stayed home. Rather than compassion, I was met with bitterness and aggressiveness. Not exactly the trip I had imagined, but I wasn't about to take sides or get involved, so kept my distance, but there was a lot of gossip going around in the little groups within the larger group trying to make sense of it all.

The day finally arrived when we embarked on the most exciting part of the trip. Walking the Inca Trail was quite a journey in many ways. Walking in the footsteps of such a magnificent culture was humbling, seeing the storage huts they built along the way that were once filled with supplies for travelers.

We hiked the trail over three nights and four days with our guide having been specially chosen as per the request for someone spiritually awake and aware. A long bus ride took us from our hotel to the starting point of the trail where we presented our passports and yellow fever vaccination proof. We then embarked on an interesting few days in close proximity. We had sherpas who carried the heavy bulky luggage – tents, sleeping bags, dining equipment, kitchen equipment – while we carried our personal belongings in our backpacks.

Our days consisted of early wake-up calls with a bowl of warm water and washcloths along with coca tea delivered to our tent entrance. We then dressed and packed our sleeping bags and backpacks and headed to the meal tent where a delicious and nutritious breakfast awaited. Warm porridge was my favourite, but the culinary skills of these humble Peruvians were outstanding. Once our meal was completed, we were on our way "vamos vamos!" being the call of our guide, telling us to hurry up. We heard this call several times through the day as some lagged behind too long taking in the scenery.

With stops for morning tea, lunch and afternoon tea giving us time to refuel and rest our bodies, we would arrive at the next campsite to do it all over again. We received information about the lives of the Inca's all along through our trek, and walking in their footsteps seemed surreal, and we definitely felt a beautiful energy walking through these incredible mountains. We saw many supply huts along the way which were built long ago by the Incans so that those journeying would always be able to renew their food along the way. Many significant spiritual sites provided us beautiful places to meditate and draw upon the ancient energy. Gaia, Mother Earth or Pacha Mama as she is fondly referred to in Peru has a preeminence with the people of this land. She is revered and honoured daily and openly for the riches she provides, and this is telling in the historic sites we visited.

I didn't find the trek easy at all. I had been still reeling from energy-zapping anaemia and it had left me with not much stamina, so I would become tired quite quickly which was disappointing for me. Coming from a background where my fitness levels had been very high and I had a resting heart of 38, it was disheartening to be exhausted from simply walking. I was hard on myself but had to keep reminding myself that there was altitude involved and that would have had a factor in the fatigue as well. The highest point of the trek was Dead Woman's Pass at 4215 metres, which is 1800 metres higher than the altitude of Machu Picchu. The altitude creeps up on you, and it is in-discriminatory as far as fitness levels and health are concerned. Some find it crippling, and some cope very easily regardless of their background. One step at a time is the mantra that is best adopted when it hits, since it can be crippling if allowed to fester.

On our final day we rose hours before dawn so that we could ascend into the Sun Gate at dawn. This is such a crucial element of the trek, as there is a steep ladder leading to the final peak which, when stepped onto, opens up the most breathtakingly magnificent vista of the ancient civilisation of Machu Picchu. It is here that we stopped for a rest and to take in the view, the energy and the magic, and to congratulate ourselves and each other on the completion of the trek. That wasn't the end by a long shot though, there was still a couple of hours to descend along the path before finally arriving at the ruins itself. When arriving we re-grouped and then spent the next several hours being guided through the history and the stories that have been pieced together by the historians and exploring the wonders of this ancient site.

Two distinct energies aligned themselves to me while I was there. Ela and Aquela-a are the names I was given, a male and female, husband and wife, soulmates with an extreme bond of deep love who have since helped me with the alignment of my inner masculine and feminine. It's like I have embodied their essence in mine. The feeling is that of a deep supported love, and when I meditate with their energy it is warm and palpable, like a big hug from heaven. They continued to be with me in spirit for a few years after this experience, guiding my journey many times.

As our trip came to an end, we all resumed our lives with the added dimension of all that this trip had given us. Like anything worthwhile, it's the journey itself that brings us our greatest gifts, it's the lowest lows that beckon us to take those difficult steps into the next chapter, lighter and clearer in our direction with each undulation that we explore. We must leave things and people behind, we must restrict the energy suckers in our life, the friends who drain us and don't give back, the situations at work where we feel like we are selling our souls in return for money, the things we spend money on to fill our life with purpose, the people pleasing, the escapism when we see ourselves as a victim of our circumstances, the blaming and shaming, the guilt trips, the self-pity, the old stories we cling to as excuses for being angry, bitter and unforgiving.

There was a niggling internal voice telling me that I needed to have a session with my teacher. It was so strong that I followed up and made the call to book the session. She reluctantly booked me in and on the day, there was tension in the air as I followed her into her room. As the session began, she felt it necessary to tell me exactly what she thought I should be doing, all from a perspective of anger and aggression. I felt like walking out because she wasn't conducting the session professionally but getting all caught up in her ego and opinion. As I sat silently, praying she would just get on with things, she finally allowed a deeper connection, softened considerably as she channeled through some deep wound issues coming up around me and asked me to lay on the massage table to check my body for blockages and messages.

As the next 20 or 40 minutes or more unfolded, the energy that was running through my body caused me to pulsate up and down aggressively on the table, sit bold upright at times, and feel a lead weight bear down upon my body as she worked into and around my energy centres.

It was the most aggressive energetic healing I have ever had, and it left her sobbing on the floor, mascara running down her cheeks and apologising for being so rude to me. She had seen something during that healing that took her to another level in herself, while disarming the attacking manner she had with me. It was humbling to see her like this.

To this day I'm not sure who got more out of that session, but I think it was her. On some level I believe we all help each other, and while I was well on my journey by now, we as healers needed to support each other in our own growth. 'The student becomes the master' seems an adequate way to look at this course of events.

After this, I felt such gratitude for everything she had brought to my life. The initial awakening, the teaching of kinesiology, the gentle persuasion to own my gifts and higher potential, and for literally turning my life around in a way I would never have dreamed or conjured. I wanted to show her my gratitude by supporting her centre so I asked my sister to join me on the open day for her new space. We drove out together and I was excited to introduce her to my friends and show her this beautiful place and all it had to offer. We only intended to purchase a few items from her shop but as we chatted to her sister at the reception desk, she invited us to join in the crystal bowl meditation class that was due to begin but was running behind and hadn't yet started. I was reluctant because I didn't want to join in late and be disruptive, but she assured us it was all okay, just go in and grab a mat, set up, there was still plenty of time.

So that's what we did and just as we were settling down, my teacher looked over in my direction asking who was arriving late – yes there were still others settling – and proceeded to call out my name and say, that's so typical of you Carmel, late and disruptive.

It was definitely time for me to say goodbye – for good. We stayed for the class, but I didn't set foot into her centre again.

About two years later I did send her an email. I told her I wanted to convey my gratitude for all she had done, even though things had ended the way they did. I didn't think I would receive a response because that's not why I sent it, however I did. It came from a place of grace. She said that she had never witnessed someone grow as much as I had or possess the gifts that I did. She felt threatened and didn't know exactly how to direct me, hence her erratic behaviour. She conveyed that she was ashamed of her behaviour and thought I was angry with her.

How ironic that she didn't understand that I held her on the highest pedestal of all for a long period of time, which was always going to end badly. The truth is, she was one of my greatest teachers and I was honoured to be around her for the few years I needed to be. Without her, I would not have had the courage to own my greatest gift, my genius and the most divine aspect of my soul. It was fitting that we part ways with grace, respect, honour and gratitude for each other.

SIXTEEN
THE FLOODGATES OPEN

The next couple of years unfolded like a dream. My client list grew and grew. I was seeing people back to back on some days and getting referrals simply through word of mouth. Often, I saw every member of a family, many clients often referred relatives and friends to me, I was living with such love and divine purpose – something I had never experienced at such an intense level of awareness. I had thought that my greatest purpose on this earth was to be a mother and bring my four wonderful children into this world, and here I was being shown another equally important role, one that would unfold once my children were developing their own paths.

One of my friends who is a gifted psychic medium had a session with me after hearing about my abilities. This was when we had only just met, and she told me she had been seeing a healer for years until he had passed on a couple of years earlier. After her session she was astounded that she had found someone who truly was a healer. No one else had been able to heal her physical body the way he had, until now. I never cease to be amazed at the results of my healing sessions. I don't go into a session thinking I'm going to miraculously heal this person, I simply allow everything to unfold as it needs and when the time is right, the intensity picks up and we are taken into a deeper energetic space where the language and sounds flow from me, and the energy from my body transfers to theirs.

Our friendship grew and we shared many hours together talking about our experiences, but the best part was that we just sat and allowed spirit to communicate through us. It's like we threw tea parties for the spirits and we all just had a blast, seeing visions, hearing messages and overall being who we really were and feeling free to share everything we experienced.

One Saturday afternoon after our client sessions were complete, we sat and relaxed over a cup of tea. It was a beautiful day, and the afternoon sun was streaming in the back glass doors. Then Jenni laughed and said that there was a little girl spirit in front of us, she was smiling and holding out the hem of her circular dress and doing a little dance for us. I felt her presence too, and then she left the room, beckoning for us to follow her. She led us into where Daniel was playing a computer game in the next room. We asked Daniel if he could see anyone around him and he said, as if it was plainly obvious, that yes of course, he could see the little girl next to him. Then I suddenly knew exactly who she was. My little girl!

In 1998 I had a miscarriage at around four to six weeks gestation. I hadn't realised I was pregnant at the time though since I didn't track my cycle and when I had a period it was only very light and short lived. I was on the pill at the time so falling pregnant wasn't on my radar.

Andrew and I had been in the city and were walking through a large department store when I felt very sharp and intense cramps, again something uncommon for me. I thought I might be getting my period. I thought I'd be okay, but they became worse, and I had to find somewhere to sit down while Andrew went to a pharmacy for some pain relief for me. While I was sitting and waiting, I needed to use the bathroom. Luckily there was one nearby and it was there I passed blood, which looked unlike my usual period, but I didn't take too much notice at the time. After that I took the paracetamol and when I felt a little better, we continued walking again slowly.

The next day I felt normal again and I hadn't continued bleeding as I would have for a normal period. It was several years before I realised I had a miscarriage that day.

So, here she was! The little girl who was still with us in spirit, showing us she was indeed around! I told Jenni this and she asked if I had ever given her a name, which I had not. She encouraged me to give her a name since that's what she was wanting, and so I said that since Ryan would have been named Sophia, I would love to name her that. As we were talking about this, Daniel looked at us and told us that she was very happy to be called Sophia. Daniel was unperturbed with his spiritual sister beside him, as if she was no stranger to him. Jenni told me Sophia was just so happy to be around us and it was time she revealed herself. She loved being around Daniel in particular.

What a day that was, she brought so much beautiful energy into the home and it was heartening to know the bond my two little ones shared. Over the coming weeks Daniel revealed that Sophia often walked to and from school with the boys. Once they were in the classroom – and this is the best part – she then spent the day playing with the other child spirits that were also around the school.

During the course of the following year, the connection with Jenni slowly dwindled and our time together came to an end. We had come together for a greater purpose and it was now running smoothly and had grown a life force of its own. It was time we both moved on in our own directions once more. I don't fear losing friends like this, since I've had so many wonderful friends in my life whom I no longer see. The saying that people come into your life for a reason, a season or a lifetime is one that I often refer to. I believe we all have soul contracts, and we should look upon our time together as a blessing, since we never know how long we will be in each other's lives. Often one person needs the connection more than the other, but it all balances out.

I had been running weekly meditation classes since the very early days after my trip to Peru. Quite a following developed on a regular basis as people recognised that my special take on meditation included channelled messages and healing energy for everyone in the room.

As my vocabulary of spiritual language increased and my toning became more mature, the environment created within the room was other worldly. I wanted to have an approach of openness and respect from everyone in the room and encouraged sharing any relevant feelings regarding our meditation in the ten or more minutes after we finished.

Many people began sharing of their visions, colour bursts that appeared, hearing messages, seeing images and all manner of experiences they had in the session. This was a safe place to talk openly and without judgment, knowing that many people can't talk about their spiritual experiences to their close family for fear of being considered a bit psycho or deranged. I've actually been labelled as deranged by a close family member, so I know what that feels like.

Somewhere along the way a I became aware that the purpose of my weekly meditations was not what I wanted it to look like. There was gossip and complaining entering into the sacred space, even directly after the session. I noticed people took advantage of this open space to begin airing their problems and grievances. I felt uncomfortable, and reinstated that conversation be limited to the experiences inside the session.

Perhaps I was a little late though and had let this go on for too many weeks and some regulars dropped off, they were sick of hearing the same low vibe conversation from the same people. It was definitely a lesson for me to hold higher standards in my sacred space. It wasn't long before I cancelled both of my weekly classes simply because I wanted to break the cycle, cleanse the energy and maybe begin again in a few weeks or months.

Since then I have run weekly meditation classes for long periods of time, with breaks of sometimes a few weeks or months. The work I do and the energy it requires must be respected and honoured, and that only comes from a place of respect and honour within, and I always feel when the time is right to begin or to pause the classes.

Along with seeing clients for spiritual healing and transformation, I also worked part time as a Pilates instructor at a private studio. I had been working in the fitness industry since the birth of my first child when I was 24 and had recently trained to be a teacher of Pilates, both mat and reformer.

Reformer Pilates uses apparatus to provide resistance and is wonderful for building strong lean muscle mass and also for rehab, injury prevention of general fitness and wellbeing. I had only ever taught high energy classes during the 20 plus years prior, along with doing personal training and running weight loss programs with great success. The change of pace felt right, and Pilates was great for my body too. So, when an opportunity came up to work at a health club only 2.5 kilometres from home I took it. I hadn't been actively looking but it felt right.

I quickly went from teaching three classes a week to six, then ten and over the next few years I got up to teaching over twenty classes a week. In hindsight, I'm not sure how my focus shifted from doing mostly healing work, to doing mostly Pilates teaching since it seemed subtle and gradual. I was still seeing clients which I don't ever want to stop doing, however there was a shift taking place.

In late 2018 it was time to review my life and listen to the messages within which were presenting through feelings of great fatigue. I knew something was going on and a shift was due. I knew I had to walk away from some of my classes, but I loved each and every one, it was so hard to decide which ones to withdraw from. It took me six months, and during this time I became even more fatigued – not knowing why – but I eventually decided to cut out all of my evening classes. I thought this would be a step forward and I would address the fatigue, while also focusing on my healing work.

The hours that I freed up by doing this created time and lots of it. I was still very fatigued, even though I was teaching only half of my classes, which seemed odd. Even though I now had so much more time to focus on my clients and my healing business, I became what I felt was lazy and bored, and even mildly depressed in that downtime. It wasn't that I didn't want to be active and creative, I simply didn't have the wherewithal to even construct my days in a way that promoted excitement and satisfaction.

A few weeks into this time I was presented with a Facebook post that caught my eye by an author coach. I was intrigued. I love writing and have been posting blogs on my Instagram and Facebook page for a few years. Writing a book seemed like a good idea, one that I had tossed around quite a bit over the years too. I reached out and connected to Dawn Bates via a call and purchased her two-month course on the spot.

It was an intense, deep and profound journey into not only writing, but everything that could possibly arise when taking this course of action. It certainly contained the guidelines and steps required to write a successful book, but the majority of the time on those calls was spent deep in counselling, in diving deep into my old wounds that would potentially destroy my chances of writing and publishing this book. What came up was mind blowing for me. Together we journeyed through all my important relationships and how they affected my behaviour. Together we laughed and cried as I blurted out stories I had held inside for too long that were delaying another part of me to unfold. Stories that captured and held onto shame, abandonment, dependency, grief and guilt.

Week by week I grew freer of my inhibitions and I began writing.

There were questions: What should I include, what should I leave out, who will judge or criticise me, will anyone even read my book? Who am I to even write a book? Is it a silly idea? Then again many of my clients have all encouraged me to write one. This process can inhibit all creativity, yet it's only human to ask all of these questions, especially considering my book was autobiographical to a large extent, even though the primary focus was on my spiritual journey. I decided to just begin writing and see where it took me.

After working on my manuscript, diving deeply into many memories and stories, some of which were difficult to write about, I began finding it difficult to continue. Then I woke up one morning, opened my computer and my entire manuscript was gone. Completely gone. Unable to be located anywhere. I was shocked, but on a deeper level I was relieved. I knew deep in my gut that there was another way to write this book, and that the lost manuscript was exactly where it was meant to be. It had drawn some deep emotional wounds to the surface where I had spent hours working through issues from the past and found a way to move forward from them. It had been a cathartic healing experience for me, and I would eventually get this book written. Those ten thousand words had been my warmup.

Reading this book is a testament to the fact I did go on to complete it, however during the course of writing it, I went through some major upheavals and had some amazing revelations. I will go into this in detail in another chapter since it carries great significance.

SEVENTEEN
EGYPT 2015

It was time. Egypt had been calling me, I listened to her. I was being summoned to a spiritual awakening and joined a tour which I knew would be perfect. I chose a tour based on it being a spiritual pilgrimage and was drawn to a woman who had been on many journeys alone, and with groups. She teamed up with Ahmed, a sixth generation Egyptologist who lives and breathes not only the factual and evidence-based history, but in recent years had embraced a deeply spiritual aspect since honouring his calling to connect to his soul voice. He grew up literally in the backyard of the Pyramids of Giza, with his father and grandfather teaching him their wisdom from a very young age.

Our small group of seven travelled to Aswan, Upper Egypt, to begin our three-week journey of this land of mystery, choosing to travel for 36 hours straight rather than have an overnight stay somewhere. We could then take a couple of days to recover before beginning our real journey, the inward one. Our first hotel was in Aswan where we rested and recovered from the long haul and began easing our way into the culture, the climate and the time zone.

We then began exploring some sites and villages before embarking on the main attractions, one of which being the temple of the goddess Isis, Philae temple. I was excited about this since I had been drawn to the

Goddess Isis for some time and felt a deep connection with her energy. Our day began with a 3.30am wake up call, we began the trek by bus and boat so that we would arrive in time for sunrise. As I dressed that morning, I knew that I wanted, was feeling called to, dress in all white. It was on the bus that I began feeling a cosmic sensation in my body, a floating sensation encompassing my entire body and expanding my heart space, I could literally feel my chest rise and expand as I invited the full intensity of this preparation work to integrate on all levels of my being. I became distant, silent, introspective. A journey had begun as the distance between the temple and I contracted.

The boat ride to the island was the final leg of the trip. I stood the entire way just taking in the magnificence of the sight before me. We stepped off the boat and Ahmed led us into the grounds. I seemed to float as we made our way to the rooms inside the main building. One of these rooms was where the inner sanctum of Isis was located, with a stone altar about the size of a lectern in the centre of the room. As I entered, I felt an overwhelming upheaval of emotion. I walked around the room, taking in the hieroglyphics, placing my hand in the well-worn place inside one wall that we were shown. It was a ritual of old that bestowed blessings on each person whose hand rested there. And then we made our way to stand around the altar as Ahmed began to teach us the history of this sacred space in his own words, from the knowledge handed down to him, and in combination with his own spiritual connection and beliefs.

During the entire time I was holding in a tidal wave of emotion. Yet I remained in my own inner world of wonder, bliss and super-overwhelm, unable to convey to anyone the enormity of my internal spiritual eruption. Then, as Ahmed spoke, I let out a howling sob, and continued to uncontrollably break open lifetimes of feminine empowerment and knowing, as the Goddess called me to release lifetimes of inherited clutter here in her inner sanctum, formally activating our Divine connection. I lost my legs and fell to my knees, bowing to the ground in raw and primal, wild woman liberated freedom. There I stayed and allowed all of the shame to rise up and out of me, the guilt and suppression from lifetimes lived, having bottled up who I am, what I came for. I let it go, the clinging to restrictive beliefs and behaviours that kept me chained to pain and grief, for the shrinking and defeated healer that was literally dying to live, time and again.

Isis held me. She embraced my inner child as the loving and divine nurturer that she is. She held my heart in those moments, for it was tender and breaking open as I died a thousand deaths for all the suppressed women before me.

I took the time I needed, and Ahmed graciously led the rest of the group away to give me space. I then made my way around the temple in silence, integrating the ongoing process inside of me. I was led by Ahmed into another room where he knew I needed to be. As I began to feel into this room and embody the energy in the hieroglyphics, my body was automated like it had been so many times in recent years, and I began circling the room, channeling the ancient ones in their tongue, toning deeply intense notes and singing the words of Isis. The peace and deep, deep love this imbued in my heart was profound, beyond words. There was one hieroglyphic that drew my gaze with each rotation, two hands joined, lovers. Over and over my gaze held this image until finally I stopped and stood in front of it, singing the most magnificent song of love, tears streaming down my face with such depth of emotion.

I held her energy as mine until it no longer felt separate. I know this energy is not one to be confined or defined, but rather it is to imbue so that it may then radiate outward to all who desire it through my work and my life.

EIGHTEEN

THE NILE CRUISE

A four-day Nile cruise followed soon after this experience. I was looking forward to feeling the flow of the Nile beneath me as I slept at night, hoping for dreams that would whisper the secrets of Isis to me. It all began beautifully as we settled into our cabins. When we weren't moving along the Nile, we spent the days docked and had the opportunity to wander the local streets of Upper Egypt with their street markets and coffee houses. We spent many hours at these cafes enjoying Egyptian coffee and refreshments.

My absolute favourite food while in Egypt was the casual meals in these cafes. The fresh warm flat bread with the most divine assortment of dips made with the freshest of ingredients, and the warm ta'meyya, the Egyptian name for falafel filled flatbread sandwiches that melted in my mouth. I also purchased dried Hibiscus flowers to bring home with me after learning the correct method for making this delicious tea.

We visited a Nubian village where time seemed to have stood still. We were welcomed to wander around and chat to the villagers before sitting with them and enjoying refreshments and photos. We also watched them baking bread for a feast the following day which I found a fascinating process. The women worked in a tiny kitchen where the temperature was almost unbearable for hours on end. I asked Ahmed if he could arrange for us to purchase a loaf of this bread to bring back to the boat with us for afternoon tea.

Back on the boat we sat on the top deck by the pool and drank tea and enjoyed the bread dipped in rich molasses, it was delicious. Before long I became frustrated with the conversation in the group and left to go down to my cabin where I felt tired so had a rest until it was dinner time. I felt a bit off and didn't eat much before excusing myself early and going to bed. During the night I became quite ill with a stomach bug, racing to the bathroom to evacuate everything I had consumed, from both ends.

In the morning I called and said I wouldn't be visiting the planned sights today and would instead rest and get over this bug. I slept and drank water all day, but my stomach was still very uneasy. When I tried to eat something that evening it didn't stay down, so I spent another night in and out of the bathroom. The next morning, I let them know I wouldn't be attending the tours once again and by this time I was feeling very weak. Some of the group came to visit me to see if there was anything they could do but I told them I just needed to rest. My beautiful tour friend did some energy healing on me as well. The following morning, I really wanted to try to get up and go on the tour, but after going to the bathroom I felt very dizzy. As I put my foot down on the step to exit the bathroom, my legs went to jelly and my head began spinning. Down I went, banging into the confined walls like a bouncy ball several times on the way to the floor. This was the morning of the third day since I fell ill. I had spent all that time in my cabin trying to recover but getting worse.

That evening I finally asked to be taken to the doctor, and Ahmed immediately arranged priority treatment at a clinic about twenty minutes' drive away. Although the town was in quite a primitive part of Egypt, the medical facilities were fantastic. The doctor immediately did an ultrasound and blood test from a prick in my finger. Through these he determined the strain of bug I had and prescribed medication. We left in the waiting car and proceeded to the pharmacy where he picked up a large bag which contained all of my medication. Next stop, to my surprise was the local public hospital. Why are we here? I asked. You need some needles, he replied.

Again, he pulled strings and I was quickly admitted to a bed in a ward ahead of many others standing around both inside and outside the hospital doors. We were led to a ward with several small vinyl beds, badly in need of repairs, one of which I laid down on, and very soon a nurse attended to me. She reminded me of Florence Nightingale, a pristine crisp white uniform of slacks and coat and hijab, smart and beautiful, quickly attending to finding out what I needed. She returned about 30 minutes later since the hospital was very busy and I was lucky to be given such special treatment. She tied a surgical glove around my lower arm to find a vein – no fancy equipment here – and proceeded to place the cannula in the back of my hand, ready to receive the drip. She also jabbed my butt with one or two more injections, then another one or two went into the saline solution on the drip stand. By this stage I was so dehydrated it was all I could do to just watch what was going on and follow simple instructions, however I had my tour guide with me every single moment for support, and thanks to him I felt as safe as I would in my own home.

The first drops entering my veins felt like the cool river of life flowing into my parched veins. Words cannot describe that feeling of pure bliss as I lay in complete surrender and trust. After the first bag there was another and I realise now that I must have been given the thickest sized needle so as to quicken the process. I don't know how long we were gone, but I do know that if I didn't receive treatment that night, I would most likely have been found unconscious in my cabin before much longer. The nurse would not take the money discreetly offered to her by Ahmed, she smiled and told him she was just doing her job. But we all knew she had moved small mountains to attend to me so expediently. We were driven back to the ship where I had a sound night's sleep of recovery. By the next morning I was ready to begin exploring again, I had missed three days of our tour, and several temples and sites.

Knowing that this sojourn to Egypt was of a deeply spiritual nature, I knew that my energy would be restored for the places I needed to visit, that my soul needed to visit. And so, it was that my next incredible experience was in the temple of Dendera, the temple of the goddess Hathor. This large and extremely well-preserved temple held more of the magical essence of the Divine Goddess I was now embodying. It was after the initial tour, and as I was wandering around, that I was drawn to walk down the large stairway. The story goes that Hathor would prepare herself for the return of her husband Horus, the son of Isis and Osiris, when he returned from his long journeys. Theirs was a love of epic proportion, and upon his arrival she would glide down the stairs, filled with joy upon his safe return.

As I stood at the top of the stairway, its walls spilling with magnificent hieroglyphs, I felt her presence, her absolute joy, the deepest love and affection and the anticipation. I made my way down feeling into this experience and knowing that my soul was communicating with her soul. This stairway was a portal of divine love. I knew that as I had once again dressed in all white on that morning, this would be a visit to not only remember, but to remain in my heart and soul, expanding the feminine codes within. This temple had seven rooms depicting the journey through the seven chakras or energy centres. Beginning with the base chakra located at the base of the spine, we had the opportunity to spend time in each of the chambers to feel into the energy and perhaps allow a healing process to take place, clearing stagnant energy from these centres. I loved this journey, moving from the base through to the sacral, solar plexus, heart, throat, third eye, and finally emerging into a much larger room to complete the journey of healing (for now), arriving at the crown chakra, located at the top of the head. Just like at the Philae temple of Isis, I experienced long stretches of time where I felt surreal and other worldly.

When I arrived back at my hotel, I rested for a few moments before being beckoned from within to dance a dance of commitment. The way my body moved in a mix of ballet, ballroom and sacred dance movements felt delectable. I was an embodiment of the divine feminine essence as I entered another realm, once again into a place where time and space didn't exist, gracefully flowing into every step, feeling the meaning behind many of the moves, stepping into and out of parts of me, embracing the inner wild woman, letting go of the oppressed keeper of the codes since they no longer needed protection. I was now embodying these codes which would continue to work their way through me over the coming months and years. During that dance of devotion, I have never felt so held, loved and honoured so utterly and completely, yet so free and empowered. I have never felt so safe and seen, deep into my soul. Time was of no significance, nor was language, I danced through time and space like it was eviternity – the space where angels reside. I was one. I was embodied with the purest essences of love in sacred union, like the image in the hieroglyph of the intertwined hands at Philae temple.

My heart was so full it was overflowing, I was light and free of the heavy weight of doubt, shame and loneliness. I danced into the answers to my questions, the answers to my longing for more. I danced my way home, and my heart would never be the same again. Chambers in my heart which were once closed off, being thrown open once more, freeing me from the fear of hurt, pain and suffering. As they opened, light poured in to eliminate the shadows of suffering and illusion, and delusion. The delusion I had been living that had kept me feeling like I was a failure, that there was something wrong with me, questioning why I couldn't fit into the norms of relationships and life like everyone else did, getting itchy feet, feeling unfulfilled, wanting more but not knowing what that was, ultimately leading to my deepest longing for answers. Like Aladdin, I had freed my own genie.

NINETEEN
KUNDALINI RISING

On the flight from Luxor to Cairo, heading into the final week of our trip, I found myself in conversation with the man sitting next to me. It wasn't long before we realised we both had a passion for exploring the spiritual side of our world, and our conversation began exploring depths that cannot be reached with just anyone. My intuition was telling me via deep vibrations in my stomach – my creative/sexual centre – that this is no chance meeting, it has been divinely orchestrated at the perfect moment. Having experienced the embodiments of divine goddess energy over the prior two weeks, I was ready to embody the essence of a similarly awakened masculine. Not some inconsequential dalliance, but a heart-hurtling and intense dive deep into the very vibration of union on the physical plane, accompanied by the awareness of the soul unity - creating the perfect hallowed ground for the dance to come.

The experience in Philae when I was mesmerised by the image of the two hands depicted in the hieroglyph, the one I was magnetically drawn to, wept into and sang the vibrations of a higher consciousness into, was now making sense. Each time I re-live the experience of that moment, my entire womb space dances, like a child inside the womb. It's my sign of a creative force beckoning me to trust the next steps I am guided to take, not second guessing and questioning them and procrastinating, as has been my pattern in life. You see, even though I often jump into life at the deep end, when I think too much, when I see that I can achieve so much more than I ever thought possible, that's when I fall down into a pit of doubt and fear. Fear of rising into more than I know how to be, or how to handle. That fear keeps me locked down in the quicksand of my uncomfortable comfort zone, my discomfort zone. Try as I might, and I have tried to overcome this so many times in my life, I just can't climb out, that growth-averse density drags me down with its many voices ready to explain just why I should stay put, stay small.

> The voices say:
> "You'll never be able to sustain that level even if you do reach it."
> "What would you possibly know about living a life so different to the one you're living now?"
> "If you rise to that next level of mastery in your life, and if you dare to claim money, earned by living the life of your lofty dreams, doing what you know you are here to do, how can you justify it?"
> "What about all those who will suffer from your gain?"
> "Leave it to the ones who know how to do it right, the ones who deserve to be there."

Yet here I was, experiencing that feeling, knowing there was something larger for me than my obscured vision of the world allowed me to think, unfolding in these precious moments. We were stuck there whether we liked it or not, on a plane that had us sitting very close, unable to avoid moments of uncomfortable yet unquestionable connection.

The vulnerability soon lead into trust. The immediate trust you have in finding a common thread, a thread that for you has grown into a steely rope inside your soul, entwining itself again and again, growing in strength and experiences. It was obviously time for another thread to be added to this now strong and unbreakable steel cable. It was up to both of us to allow and invite the weaving to begin. He happened to be staying at the same hotel as our group was in Cairo, and so we met for coffee and had more in-depth conversations over the course of the week.

On the next morning after arriving in Cairo we met again, he was sitting on the opposite side of the large foyer in the hotel cafe, at least 30 meters away. I spotted him chatting to others and made my way over to say hello. Then something strange happened. I lost all stability in my spine and began collapsing to the floor. I managed to find my footing before I completely fell but I went to jelly, not in my legs, in my spine.

It wasn't long before I realised what had happened. My spine was and is very healthy and strong, so it was nothing physically, that is to say there was nothing physically rooted in the reason behind the collapse.

In the moment that it happened, I felt a very strong bolt of energy shoot from my tailbone right up my spine. It wasn't painful in the least; it was purely potent energy running through my body. This happened again and again over the next three days, each time I saw this man, it kicked off a spark that ignited me again and again until the process was complete. It was nothing sexual, even though our sex centres were definitely being ignited, it was the raw and deeply primal contact between two souls who were destined to meet to share something they were both ready for. He also received an energetic burst from being in my presence and it was beyond wonderful to be able to talk openly about our experiences in wonder, and in gratitude to each other.

He told me that since we met, something inside of him knew it was destined to be. While he didn't experience the kundalini/spinal charge that I did, he experienced something equally deep within his soul knowing. He felt like we had known each other in some other dimension and were now meeting in the flesh in this physical dimension. He told me that he felt such a familiarity with me that he could immediately indulge in conversations that he could have with no one else. We felt like we were married souls.

We met after dinner each evening over the following days and would sit by the pool with the familiarity of lovers, relating our life stories to each other. On a couple of those nights we drove around the city of Cairo and its outskirts just so we could spend more time together. We would stop at cafes and drink tea and relate more of our desires and just chat about everyday life on different sides of the world. It wasn't a steamy lustful feeling, more of a slow burn that didn't require an urgency or a destination.

Over these five days I went on several tours to the Great Pyramid and the surrounds, visiting an oil fragrance factory where I purchased some beautiful fragrances including jasmine, lotus flower and white lotus, which I still use sparingly five years later. It is in these factories that the base for the world's famous fragrances like Chanel No.5 are derived and exported. We also visited the home of our guide Ahmed's grandparents, a home in which he spent a great deal of time growing up and learning the traditions of Egyptology. The hospitality we received was very warm and welcoming. We were invited into their home as guests and served refreshments while we chatted to our hosts about everything Egyptian history.

At this stage of the trip I felt like winding down after experiencing such highs in the temples we visited while staying in Luxor. Our group was beginning to become a little disjointed too which I guess is normal after spending almost three weeks together in often confined spaces. Personalities were clashing and it brought back memories of my Peru trip. It's funny how some people just want to remain in a position of power and when they feel threatened in their position as leader of a group they want to stomp out any hint of losing their power.

To elaborate, it became obvious to a few in our group that my gifts were becoming disruptive to our tour leader (not Ahmed). It began early in our tour when I sang the enchanted song in the Abu Simbel temple and was hushed by our tour leader. Then a few days later at dinner I was asked to channel a blessing by my new lovely friend and co-tour participant who I had come to really like, she's just gorgeous. She was right next to me in the temple and was just dying to hear that voice again. All eyes were on me and I felt a little self conscious since I wasn't sure what I was going to bring forth. Then I closed my eyes, took a breath and began singing a beautiful song of activation to bring forth blessings for all present. It must have lasted at least one minute, which is a long time, but I was completely lost in the euphoric feeling enveloping me as I brought forth this blessing song. It is always a reverent experience for me and takes me far away and into a place of complete surrender, and I usually beam with a beautiful big smile while singing.

It became obvious to my new friend that our tour leader was a bit jealous or something because, even though I offered to lead a meditation for our group and the others loved that idea, she didn't want me involved at all. It seemed I was stepping over a line that she wanted me to remain firmly behind and in my place as a participant in her group. Now when we were travelling as a group to our outings there seemed to be more distance between us. I guess that's only natural after three weeks together though, however it would seem that I tend to test people while being in complete integrity with myself. And now we were on the final days of the countdown to the end of our epic tour.

The final night approached all too quickly. We both knew this serendipitous union of souls in bodies was coming to an end. We wanted to do something special on our last evening. He would arrange everything.

With his connections and in total respectful secrecy, we were picked up and driven to a small village about 20 minutes away. I still didn't know what was arranged, and as we slowed, parked the car and alighted, I saw a man walking towards us leading three horses behind him.

"Can you ride?" He asked me.

"Yes, but it's been a long time," I answered.

Introductions were made and we mounted our horses. My long black flowing dress, scarf and sandals were the perfect attire for this storybook moment. Then our guide lead us out of the village and into the most beautiful desert sands where we rode, walking and galloping over dunes, until we reached a point, secluded but still within distance of other freedom seekers, mostly locals, riding on the grounds of the ancient spirits who once roamed these deserts. I laid my scarf down on the sand and we sat, looking out to the three majestic pyramids in front of us. It was like we could reach out and touch them. This private work of art lay before us, emanating love and mystery, ancient knowing and the blessings of gods and goddesses upon us. It was in sheer reverence we sat, and then lay, taking in the skyscape of diamonds above us.

Mesmerised as we were with the sheer holiness of the moment, the absolute comfort of lying in each other's arms, we kissed, sealing this moment in our respective and unified souls forever. I have never experienced anything so absolutely divine in this life. If we could capture that moment and put it in a treasure chest, it would be one that when discovered, would burst open the hearts of generations and saturate them in a love that would bring them to their knees in awe. It would be rich enough to spread, potently contagious and travel with lightning speed to heart after heart, overcoming doubt and fear, slicing through the instilled unworthiness and victimised behaviours, unblocking the eternal springs of this fierce and impassioned energy.

Kundalini. "She who is coiled." Refers to the powerful creative sexual energy coiled like a sleeping serpent near the base of the spine. One of the goals in Tantra is to gently awaken this dormant energy in order to awaken consciousness and attain enlightenment.

To this day the codes continue to be activated regularly, it's an open channel and they are available to me each time I am ready – that is, each time I take an action, make a decision or embody my spiritual essence or take the intuitive hint and put it into action to up-level my life, I am taken through another process of up-levelling, all very different but similar to the ones I experienced in Egypt. My life is filled with the healing codes of the Divine, for the explicit purpose of bringing them to all who so desire. It is my role to work with those who are ready to move into their soul journey, their unexplored potential, their untapped creativity. It is my role to show others the way to clear their energy centres of the blockages holding them back, to cut through the old stories and beliefs given to them by a lineage holding onto fear and shame, a society of control and restriction and religious beliefs that have been distorted over centuries.

I know that each time I receive these upgrades, many, many others are ready for their upgrades and that I am available to be the one who takes them through the process. It has happened countless times with many clients, and I am honoured to have followed the call of this legacy I carry. Apart from being a mother to four incredible humans, this is the one other purpose for my existence. Of this, I am certain.

TWENTY
DANCES OF INCEPTION

When I separated in 2011 it took me many months to find the confidence to step up into financial responsibility and move into my own place with my boys. When I finally made the step, I found that doorways opened up to me with such ease. I easily paid all my bills and was able to save money as well. This was such a welcome feeling of independence, a true awakening into finding what was really beneath my surface.

I found that running had been a way of inviting and enlightening my inner problem-solving skills. After a run I felt clearer, and solutions were reached where only staleness had been. I found a new running path that was fantastic, through nature for most of the way and I would go anywhere from five to eight kilometres depending on my day. I became very familiar with the path and the feeling I got in different places. Some places I ran through felt dark and dense and others felt light. Then it began. I had been clearing energy in my home and other places for months now, and it was time to take it outdoors. Sometimes on my run, I would involuntarily slow down to a stop, change direction and go off into an area that obviously had stuck and low energy, it felt dead, the trees looked dead even though they were green. Then the dance would begin, a circular spinning dance taking me within a circumference defined by my guides, always Mother speaking with me and comforting me as I would become more and more dizzy the quicker the spinning became. I felt like a spinning top weaving in and around trees at quite an intense pace. Finally, I would begin to slow and be so grateful that it was almost over, only to realise that I needed to do the exact same dance in the other direction. That was always how it happened, one direction and then the other. At the end of this process I felt so light and happy, knowing that I had shifted something that was keeping this place stale and harbouring very low state energy.

I continued to do this for quite some time and always loved running through the areas that I had worked and danced in. They were lighter and radiated a beautiful feeling as I passed. Going through these experiences has highlighted to me that we as humans, in our physical bodies, really need to do the work we are guided to, crazy as it sometimes sounds. I know that our angels are sometimes so demanding of us for the explicit reason that we need to keep our end of the relationship going. A physical body is required to complete many of the upgrades and miracles that happen every day. The only way to do this is to listen to and follow our intuition. That's crucial.

And there, is the problem for many.

What is intuition, and how is it distinguishable from a random thought? How do we know we can trust out supposed intuition, and not end up looking foolish?

The way I've learned is that it's usually something you wouldn't normally think of doing or saying. Mostly, but not always it's pretty random, and the more you just go with it regardless, stop questioning and reasoning and figuring it out, just go with the feeling you get. See what happens. Often there is no big revelation. Sometimes it might be simply talking to someone and lifting their spirits from an otherwise lonely or depressing feeling of being alone and unseen. It's a bit like our cravings for food. When we eat healthily, we usually only crave the foods our body requires for something in particular in that moment. I eat very differently depending on what season it is, and often cut out whole food groups entirely for days or weeks. Like the times I eat mostly fruit. Mangoes, kiwi fruit, bananas, berries of all kinds, pawpaw, all the tropical fruit. I practically live on it and sidestep salads and grains almost entirely. Other times I crave salads, other times roasted vegetables, sometimes mushrooms, and often combinations that I would never think of but following my craving I discover new combinations. When this happens, I know that the combination of the nutrients of the foods I just knew I had to have, is perfect for bringing my body back to a more balanced state.

Since becoming vegetarian in 2012, six weeks prior to my first trip to Peru, I have remained almost entirely vegetarian and often close to vegan. The reason I chose to become vegetarian was because it was a requirement of the spiritual journey that we all lighten our body's density by not eating the flesh of animals, which is hard not only for our physical body to digest, but for our spiritual body also. When we eat the flesh of another sentient being, we embody its DNA and so much of the pain and suffering it endured in its life, and you can imagine how much suffering that would be if an inhumane slaughtering practice was used. The living conditions, the abuse if any all of that comes into play, and as time went on, I decided I felt much better in myself not eating meat, seafood or chicken. I rarely eat eggs now since they don't sit well with me either when I do have them.

Most vegetarians and vegans supplement their diet with many different grains and pulses. I don't like them; they don't agree with me and so I rarely eat them unless I'm out and there are dishes that include them. There's also the viewpoint of eating food that's been prepared with love. This seems to be the vital ingredient regardless of the food. My mother in law is a great example, she cooks, using mostly fresh ingredients from her garden and spends time creating nutrient rich and delicious food that I just can't get enough of. I always overeat, but don't feel bloated or bad afterward, my body just craves and fills up on the love and goodness infused in her meals. When we visit, we feel like royalty, there is nothing she wouldn't do for us.

TWENTY-ONE
WORKING WITH CLIENTS

As I began working with clients in a healing capacity via channeled vibration and movement, it wasn't without doubt and a little fear. I questioned that I would somehow lose my connection and feel like a fraud and maybe learn that I had been fooling myself, that perhaps this was all just too good to be true. I mean where was my qualification, where was my teacher for what I was doing? My teacher was the Divine guidance I received. It presented like a sudden dialogue that I didn't have time to process in any way before it was being formed into the exact words to accompany the movement of energy through the body on all of it's levels – physical, mental, emotional and astral.

I am always 100% present in every way during my sessions. Having said that, I will go on to explain the sensations I feel during this time.

During my client sessions, in the capacity of healer, the transmuter of energy, the tuning fork for their vibrational frequency, I enter and become one with a higher dimension. This elevated, lofty feeling place of presence feels like I have a plethora of information available all around me, pertaining to exactly what the client with me is available to receive. In a very simplistic way of putting it, I feel like someone has joined me inside my body and I am dancing the cosmic dance of transcending trauma and pain in the most sacred techniques and moves. I feel a sense of oneness with what you might call God or source or the Divine, that feeling of complete peace yet with a plethora of knowledge and a doorway into the infinite possibilities with no sense of fear or doubt.

I cannot help but be in awe when I am in this space. Literally everything is available to me, and to my client. Resistance is the key to the puzzles of life. When resistance is called to attention and held to accountability, it begins to crumble through its lack of credibility. Being able to rise beyond the resistance of the human lack of understanding of just how I can morph so easily into this space of absolute Divine connection, has me living in the morphed condition as often as I choose.

I can go about my day and I know exactly when I'm letting go of the resistance that keeps me focussing on what is wrong in my life, what's missing in my life, how are others feeling, or perhaps judging or blaming or criticising me for this or that. When I let go of the responsibility of how another person feels about me, something magical happens. I rise to a better relationship with myself. And when I'm in a better relationship with myself, everyone benefits.

The most common scenarios I see with my clients have common threads:

- Anxiety.
- Low level chronic waves of depression.
- Suffering a physical affliction, often pain that is generalised and non-specific. Often back, neck, shoulder, knee or joint pain.
- A deep paralysing fear of action taking.
- Being stuck in a job, relationship or situation that's making them feel disconnected with themselves yet feeling compelled to stay for "all the reasons".
- Being a victim of circumstances, or simply being/feeling like a victim i.e. feeling helpless, without control.
- Being a people pleaser.
- Grieving a death or and ending or loss of some sort.
- Being unable to let go of their old stories, patterns and especially ingrained and often inherited beliefs.

I have found that self-analysis helps. Simply asking a few questions that can expand into a deeper understanding of what's going on behind the veil of symptoms that our body produces:

Do you use anxiety, stress and overwhelm as the gift that it is? Or do your best to ignore it and end up feeding it instead, only to find you are whetting its appetite for more of you.

Anxiety and stress are hungry beasts, and usually appear when you are feeling trapped, or trying to make a change, make a decision, speak your truth, stand up for yourself or try to change the circumstances around you that scare you, protect someone close to you or something that provides security for you, and/or your family.

They will consume every ounce of nutrition you provide them, for as long as you continue to provide it to them.

They are sneaky tricksters though.

They thrive on adrenalin you produce and become addicted to it.

The patterns of anxiety, stress and worry consume most of us, much of the time, and are often associated with hormonal imbalances, so it's always best to address any imbalances in the friendliest manner via herbal/natural therapies. Notwithstanding this, many often choose to medicate after being diagnosed by a "Professional", and give the all-consuming energetic leeches yet another energy to consume from us.

Often, we learn how to cope, we even learn how to bring our mind and body to a place where we feel we can release and reset. But the beast always catches onto the new practices we embody, it's the nature of the beast, the survival of the beast, and it is up to us to acknowledge, and then work with it, rather than fight it.

What if we looked at this affliction of the modern world and broke it down into a cycle that makes sense, then applied ourselves to actively navigating each aspect of the cycle.

The cycle = Stress, anxiety and worry − Creating space − Waiting − Filtering the Influx of thoughts and ideas − Taking Inspired Action via intuition − Trusting this process − Embodying the new processes, ideas and thoughts without judging them but rather observing how they feel − Feel the fear and procrastination and old patterns that begin to come up − observe this, but don't give it the driver's seat − continue this pattern until you actually make the change you have been waiting for − allow your new patterns that you have created to seed firmly – feel the onslaught of the next round of stress, anxiety and worry – wash, rinse and repeat.

Our body is our treasure map, and it holds every clue and every answer to every problem we ever have.

We usually get the clues via our physical or mental body, and often the GPS kicks in and begins navigating us to the best route to take that will lead us to the perfect solution, and often growth.

For example, a headache doesn't come from nowhere. Is it dehydration, eye strain, a tumour, or something more metaphysical like being around people or situations that are making you feel like you have a vice clamped on your temples, slowly tightening until it becomes unbearable (this one has happened to me).

A client came to me with stress around a personal situation, feeling trapped. I immediately picked up that there was an invisible umbilical cord, intact and still attached to his mother. He then told me about the hernia he had in that exact location. He went on to say how his mother was like a leech in his life, always there, always interfering, always making him feel inferior, nagging him, blaming him for the shortcomings of her other children and her husband. She was literally draining the power from his creative centre via this attachment. No wonder he and his wife weren't conceiving their own baby when this energetic force was draining his own ability to procreate.

He was scheduled for surgery the following week to remove the hernia. I advised him to acknowledge in some way, before the surgery, that in the removal of this hernia, he would also remove/release any and all energetic attachments that were connected to it.

As soon as he came out of surgery, his mother began removing herself from his life, without any influence whatsoever from him or his wife. She refused to visit him in hospital and then in the following weeks refused to even talk to him. The cord had been cut in all forms. No words, and no awkward or confronting conversations were needed. It was all taking place in the same silent way that it had been draining him.

These examples speak volumes in understanding the impact of our attachments. By breaking free from our end of an emotional trauma, we can release the tension of the belief, pattern, addiction, person or whatever may be on the other end of the connection.

This might sound harsh or impossible, or even undesirable though, when it comes to breaking free of an emotional or physical trauma when it involves removing the ties of someone close to you. From my experience personally and with clients, I know that in doing this work, it actually enhances the relationships concerned, or the relationships disappear, either gradually or suddenly. Imagine being physically restrained to another person like a Siamese twin, and then having surgery to remove the physical connection. After the surgical intervention, it doesn't mean that the twins will forever be apart and not be in each other's lives. In fact, it could mean they form an even more desirable relationship where each of them can experience the world individually and share their experiences with each other. Indeed, it might also result in them drifting apart for a short or long period, and then coming back together. Whatever happens, the freedom of attachment – forced and unhealthy attachment - will allow free will to be accessed more easily, and intuition to be followed without the restrictions of being eternally responsible for the other person/thought/thing.

Often people become very attached to being controlled or directed by another person. Over time their sense of self declines and forms very low self worth, leading to low self confidence and self esteem. These situations are commonly overridden on the outside by an exterior display of aggression, assertion, bullying and a host of power driven behaviours. This is to counteract the disempowerment on the internal level. So for example, an introvert, victim or people pleaser in the home environment can be a bully in the workplace to counteract the extreme imbalance.

TWENTY-TWO

TRUST, FORGIVENESS AND JEALOUSY

Sex and intimacy is so often the place that holds the key to relationship issues, and if I knew then what I know now, who knows what might have been.

When I entered into my last marriage with Andrew, bringing my two daughters with me, I felt a deep inner need to protect myself (and my girls) from being hurt again. After the divorce from my daughters' father, I was in a relationship for just over two years, which ended when I found out that he had been cheating on me regularly for the last year of the relationship. He denied it of course, and even though I knew it was true since I had the evidence, I forgave him and believed his tears of remorse. Everyone deserves a second chance, right? Well it didn't take long until the final blow was delivered and revealed the blatant lie he told me, with about a hundred witnesses, so I ended it for good. He still tried to claw back by offering me an overseas trip, a ring, even a baby. I grew an armour around me that was impenetrable, cold and harsh. I had zero sympathy, compassion or forgiveness for him.

When he turned up at my door with the most expensive French champagne, fresh lobster and seafood platters, I let him in, ate and drank and shared old times, then told him to leave. I didn't care that he was intoxicated, that was his problem. He had been used to getting his way for way too long with his charm and charisma. There was not one ounce of love left for him, my heart had been shattered, again – just differently this time.

What led me to this moment was that by stepping back, out of the infatuation bubble I was in, I saw the patterns he lived by. Very high highs, very low lows, and not much in between, lots of alcohol and social drugs to numb his lows and feed his highs. I always supported him during the lows, along with another woman, but I didn't know that. I knew that his previous marriage ended when he found out his wife was cheating and this is the story he held responsible for ending that marriage, but I also know that his constant cheating during the marriage – via the drunk stories he told me about all the young girls who threw themselves at him and his friends at the nightclubs – gave her every reason to look for comfort and companionship elsewhere.

It didn't take long for the fear of betrayal to arise in my relationship with Andrew. What happens if he meets someone else, what happens if I find out he's cheating, how do I protect myself from being hurt again? How can I be sure that I'll be okay if the same thing happens again? How can I protect myself and my girls and not be subjected to a shattered heart once more? I cannot possibly endure that again.

So I made a pact with myself. I would give 90% of myself to our marriage, and I would save 10% – just in case. Just in case he abandoned me, just in case he cheated, just in case my heart would be shattered again. And I lived with that escape route buried in my heart for the next 15 years. It rarely came to the surface, but it was there. I don't know if things would have been different had I not made that pact, but when we eventually did separate, it was nothing short of heart wrenching sadness and remorse that things could have been different and we could find a way to fix our marriage.

Weeks after we had separated, he noticed that my driver's licence was in my maiden name and was devastated that I had changed it back so quickly, thinking that I couldn't wait to be rid of his name. In fact, I had never changed my licence into my married name, for the same reason that I gave only 90% of myself to our marriage, I wanted to retain my own identity in some area of our union, just in case.

Be careful with the pacts and promises you make to yourself, and if you must do something like this, dig deep to find where the desire comes from. Mine came from a place of fear, and an instinct of survival. In hindsight, I would have looked more closely at this behaviour and found a way to understand it and communicate it with him. We would have worked it out together, I would probably have done some inner work of my own via counselling or an alternative healing therapy to help me understand the pattern I had created, and I would have addressed the issues of abandonment, vulnerability and deception.

It would be remiss of me to not include that I haven't exactly been an angel in the fidelity department. I don't want to be perceived as a victim, nor do I believe in karma in the way it is often interpreted. I believe that we learn as we live, and we do not have to be fearful of repercussions from our past mistakes in the form of being punished somehow as a retaliation, an eye for an eye, or making amends.

While I'm not proud of being unfaithful in the past, I do believe that it has led me to having an extremely strong yearning to understand not only what made me stray, but what instigates it in so many marriages and committed relationships. For me, it always came down to communication, or rather lack of it. I would hide my feelings, not speak up, and fall into the people pleasing habit that overrode me in every relationship I've been in. This was deeply embedded with my fear of abandonment and not being good enough, always making sure I put my partner's happiness before my own to make sure he stayed, thus burying my own so deeply that I didn't even realise I had any, I merged his into mine, I became one with his desires and dreams.

This pattern would last for quite some time, and I have uncovered that the period of time it lasted was in direct proportion to how sick my body became, trying to tell me to listen and learn from what my body was telling me, since there is always, always, always an explanation and message attached to any dis-ease or symptom in our body. Call me a slow learner, but I chose to hold onto rashes, eczema, anxiety, fatigue, anaemia, gingivitis, eye problems and gum disease for way too long before facing the deeper state of my relationships. It's like magic when changes are made, the symptoms disappear very quickly, and if they linger then there is still work to do, perhaps in other relationships or areas of my life.

But if the changes aren't made, the symptoms can worsen and develop into major health crises, which are then diagnosed and given explanations a far cry from where they actually originated. My experience tells me, do not ignore any health symptoms, look deeply into the messages behind it.

In the eight years since my marriage ended, I have explored many different emotions around sex, marriage and relationships. It wasn't enough for me to just move forward in life without exploring my own experiences, and also seeing the patterns that exist globally around relationships and sex, in all types of relationships whether it be heterosexual, homosexual, polyamorous or undefined.

With regard to fidelity, it's been interesting to learn that the most solid relationships on the exterior, have often encountered infidelity, and some of them have thrived on it. I've learned to not judge anyone for anything until you've walked a mile in their shoes, so I try to remove myself from judgment altogether, which is often difficult because we all fall into old patterns, and society thrives on judgment and criticism. As with many things in life, it's an ongoing and daily practice.

When I found myself single again in my forties, I withdrew into a place of self-sabotage with regard to the judgment on myself. I withdrew from sex completely, in all forms including self-pleasure. For 18 months. I was repelled by the thought of sex because it had caused so much confusion and pain in every single one of my long-term relationships. I pushed down all the pleasurable, happy and euphoric times of incredible love making as well as the raw, real and urgent passionate sex, which were innumerable. I felt guilty, I felt ashamed, I felt misunderstood, I felt a deep throbbing pain in my womb, I felt drained of my very life force. I blamed myself for ruining relationships, I blamed myself for running away from my problems, I blamed myself for being ruthless. I blamed myself for disrupting my children's lives, for taking them away from the family unit they had been born into, for making them endure shared parenting time and the adult world of pain, misery and fighting, of being subjected to the unbearable pain of feeling torn in two when they felt responsible and confused, or had to choose to be with one parent over the other.

The guilt was only overcome by my innate feminine desire, obligation and commitment to protect and guide my children. It was the kryptonite that brought me back time and again from despair and deep depression. They needed me, and there was no way I could convince myself otherwise, since it seemed these four humans were a gift to my soul that fed me with a love so profound, and a will to do whatever it takes to not only survive, but to thrive.

As I think back on the time before my first trip to Peru, it reminds me of how disconnected and very judgmental of myself I was. It began with my first foray back into the world of sex after being pursued for nine months by a guy I had known for a few years, and apparently had admired me from a distance. My confidence and self-esteem was pretty low when we began talking and getting to know each other better. I didn't realise there was anything more to it, and we began talking more and sharing everyday things with each other. I still didn't see that he was attracted to me, probably because he was a lot younger than me – 20 years younger – and it didn't enter my mind he was physically attracted to me when he could have been dating women his own age. He was hot, built, strong and very masculine.

Whenever he suggested actually going out for coffee, I would immediately end the conversation. We only ever chatted via text, and saw each other in passing through our work overlap, so I felt safe enough to chat with that distance between us. There were a few times he hinted at how he felt about me, and I usually diverted the conversation. I even asked him if he was interested in meeting one of my daughters and asked if that's why he was getting to know me better. He said that he didn't even know I had daughters, though he knew I had the boys. So that was out. Then another time I laughed and told him I finally figured him out, he must be gay, and just feel very comfortable around me.

No, he wasn't gay. He said, "Why can't you just get it – I think you're really hot!"

I managed to avoid meeting up or going out with him for 9 more months, and still we chatted regularly. I arrived back from Peru just before Christmas, and as I was enjoying some down time over the holiday break, I caught up with some friends to reminisce about our experiences in Machu Picchu. As we chatted, we naturally began talking about men and our dating lives. When I was asked if I was seeing anyone I laughed and said no way. Then I remembered this guy and told them that he had been asking me out, but because of the age difference I hadn't accepted, even avoided going out with him. They called me crazy and told me to just go out and have some fun! It seemed so easy, and so right, so that night I contacted him and told him I was ready to go out.

We went out the following night, and yes, it was an incredible night which just naturally ended with us finally doing something about all that sexual tension that had been building for months. I broke the drought, finally. He was everything I needed – attentive, caring, communicative, and fully into me, but without any hang ups about commitment or the complexities of life. We saw each other on and off over the next 18 months, and it was truly a blessing to go through all the old behaviours and patterns I had always had when it came to relationships.

I expected this to lead somewhere more serious because that's all I had ever experienced. I didn't just do one-night stands, I fell in love, and quickly. But this was different. I learned it was possible to not be so serious about following the rules of society or even our own past. It was fun, easy, intense, passionate and allowed us both to continue on with navigating our lives, since we were both leading busy lives with crazy hours.

One of my favourite nights together was lying outdoors under the star-studded canvas of our planet, just staring into the cosmos, with interspersed cuddles and a little conversation. It was so comfortable to just witness and hold each other in silence, mostly. I saw a shooting star and said, "Did you see that!" He didn't, he was looking elsewhere, and it was over in a flash. About 10 minutes later maybe, I have no idea of the time that lapsed, he saw one, and I missed it. It was truly a magical evening.

This was my liberation from the self-inflicted state of abstinence and back into being a fully conscious sexual and sensual woman, there's nothing like that glow that radiates post orgasmic euphoria, it goes on for days. And as I began learning more, I discovered that regular orgasm and deep sexual pleasure, with or without a partner, is the key to the creativity in our lives.

Pleasure opens the door to unexplored potential via the portal that opens when our focus is on nothing other than the highest state of pleasure we can experience. It is my view that we have been given this gift of experiencing such states of bliss to use and expand our lives in every single way possible. We can use sex and sexual pleasure to become more creative at work, to be better parents to our children, to feed our body with more pleasurable foods, to have a better relationship with money, to let go of all the sticky and stale stories we hold onto that stagnate our growth. Sex and our relationship to our own body and its yearning for pleasure is the key to as many doors as we would like to open. The more I learned about how to use sexual energy and pleasure to enhance my life, the more I was also drawn into examining the painful wounds I still carried in my body from my past experiences. They hadn't gone away, they were just waiting for me to acknowledge them, like little landmines planted that could be triggered and wreak havoc again if I slipped back into my old patterns.

My biggest patterns had been people pleasing, having an aversion to making decisions, and an inability to express my truest desires and feelings. I was much more comfortable being around people I trusted enough to make the decisions for me. I went with the flow, and occasionally got my horns out, being a Taurus and all, but for the most part I've always been a lover, not a fighter. However, being a lover also entailed not upsetting anyone else, not shining too brightly (even though I had a yearning to be seen), putting a lid on my lofty yearning to be bigger than life.

I was a true paradox and for as long as I can remember I've lived with inconsistency and ambiguity on a deep level. I followed the rules on the outside but had something inside that was bursting to get out but had no idea how to be free without disrupting the ironclad expectations that were my loudest, silent voice. When I played squash competitively, I had the ability to win a lot of the time but would throw the game when I felt cruel for making someone else lose. The closer the game, the better I played, but I just couldn't thrash someone without feeling guilty about it.

This pattern carried over into my sex life. Growing up without any sex education, like many of us have, I didn't know what I was doing. The first time I was just silent and let him finish, not showing the discomfort and pain I was in. We were together for six years and it didn't really change much from the first time, I didn't enjoy it at all, ever. Not a single orgasm. I wasn't entirely sure what all the hype was about, but then again it was the early 80s and thus pre internet days, and sex wasn't a topic of discussion with my friends. I self-pleasured, but not often. I don't remember many nights spent sitting down together just spending time alone, and I actually didn't factor in sex as a high priority in our marriage, I had no experience in it and we never ever talked about it. We didn't venture away from two basic positions or explore anything that would require open and inquisitive communication. If I said no, he didn't question me, but there was no conversation about our sex life. I guess we were probably both as shy as each other when it came to talking about sex.

When I left, it was because of the realisation I wasn't in love, I had been infatuated with everything else about him and all he had to offer the relationship, he adored me, and in that time I grew into myself in so many ways thanks to his love and encouragement, but I loathed the intimacy, or lack of. If I knew then what I know now, how different it could have been. Hindsight can derail you, so I don't go there. I was also finding myself being really attracted to other men and feeling very sexually excited. How would I ever explain this to my husband? So, I kept it in and found myself flirting quite a lot because it felt so good.

In my subsequent long-term relationships things got much better and I entered into the world of true intimacy and heightened pleasure. But then a different problem arose, since I still had my 'aversion to conflict' pattern firmly in place, which always resulted in me diverting away from any minor or major conflict and directing the conversation to a place where it was safe. It's actually a fear of upsetting the status quo, of feeling inferior because you regard someone else as superior, of feeling so scared of making waves that you agree to pretty much anything unless its life threatening or plain crazy. This, naturally leads to a deeper integration of the old patterns, it feeds the old patterns until they become so strong that you find new and innovative ways to appear strong, confident and independent, when you are really slipping deeper into an ocean of invisibility, because heaven forbid you allow yourself to shine, to be really seen. And while during this time I did have many achievements, I was always just off the mark to be the top of my game. I never achieved first place in any of my triathlon races, or any of my body shaping comps, I never started earning the big money in the network marketing company that I put so, so much time, energy and money into. It isn't that I tried really hard and just missed out, no not at all.

The way it worked is that I would get close to achieving what I believed I desperately wanted, then I couldn't bring myself to push that little extra, the bit that makes ordinary extraordinary. It was there, oh yes it was there, I felt it and all I had to do was tap into it, very easily, I had what it took in everything I did, but I just couldn't allow myself to win, to be first, or to achieve highly, so I held back. Because to win, well that would mean I would be showing off, I'd be a tall poppy and people would judge me and I would be taking something away from someone else if I took the first place or earned the big money. It was there. I just couldn't reach it. And it killed me. It drained me of so much self-esteem, I felt robbed and defeated, but knew I was the one holding the power. How on earth could I access this? Living on the edge of that can drive you crazy or take you down. Deep down, and into a state of low level, low lying depression. A depression you can live and function with, but it slowly sucks you dry, leaving you less and less to live on, because deep down you know you are giving your life force away. I wasn't going to let that happen, so I continued to fight, right up until I collapsed, with my life blood sucked dry, right into the hands of anaemia, and I've told you that story.

My outside world reflected my inner world and that included my intimate relationships.

To understand this more, I have learned that this pattern also needed support from within my intimate relationships. I would give almost all of what I had and hold back when I was in a position to express my deepest vulnerabilities and desires. When placed in these intimate moments with my partner I felt unable to access my desires, there was something blocking the way. I know now that it was my unwavering and uncompromising vow, made eons ago in another lifetime, to not shine a light on who I really am and what I really want to bring to this world, because it would cause something catastrophic and fatal to come to pass. What a load to carry around. It was pathetic really, and in my worst memories I recall feeling panic when looking at a menu, feeling pressured to make a choice that was okay, let alone being asked to choose a restaurant to eat at, or a destination for a day trip. This sounds so crazy, but I know there are so many others who have experienced this.

Sex was the perfect intimate place to continue this deception of my soul. I opened my legs instead of my heart on so many occasions to avoid being seen. I was convincing and conniving in my methods, a true mistress of chicanery to evade the showing of my soul, to avoid talking about my deeply embedded fears and secrets.

Even I didn't know what was there, buried within my own soul since it would only ever tease me that there was so much more than I knew, so I wasn't doing this deliberately, not at first anyway. I just found out along the way that pleasure is the way to a man's heart (this proves itself in tantric education, satiate him sexually to open his heart, and vice versa with women, i.e. satiate her heart and she will open fully sexually) and I went straight there for the purpose of avoidance. In doing this, I achieved a great sex life, I believed I was fulfilled and attentive, and this would continue until it didn't. But I was setting myself up for absolute devastation in my heart, I was setting the bar and the standards in pretending I was being deeply authentic in my supposed vulnerability.

It was just like my commitment to success in other areas of my life, I would give 90%, just in case. Eventually I would avoid sex, and the reason was confusing. I felt used and unseen and this made me feel sad and lonely, but I was good at putting on my mask mainly because I slipped very comfortably into it, often not even realising I had put it on. And I was the one who created this. What a misguided dialogue I had going on. It takes courage and bravery, and sometimes sheer desperation to step out of your own shadows when you have created an uncomfortable comfort zone within them.

I knew it had reached crisis point when my avoidance became so radical, that rather than show my aching heart, I would turn the other way and allow silent tears to stream down my distorted face, while continuing to make all the 'right' sounds and movements. It's shameful and painful to say this, to own this, it's also embarrassing and gravely upsetting, I was being the lead actress in my life movie where deception was a key player. However, there was one person I wasn't convincing, and that was myself. Why would I go to such lengths to hide what I was feeling? I think you get to a point of self-deception that is so convincing, it becomes your life, it takes over your identity, you grieve the old you that is buried deep down. And just like the story of the frog in boiling water, it just became used to the tiny increments that the temperature increased, it became a little more uncomfortable but it adjusted to the changes mindlessly and continuously, not questioning why things keep getting hotter, until it died, without even trying to escape, having slipped closer and closer to death so gradually and almost peacefully. I became used to concealing my inner dam of unknown emotions and living in a low-level depressed state.

The truth was, I didn't know what I wanted to express. That might sound naive or like I just don't want to talk about it, but honestly, I didn't know what I wanted, or what I didn't want, or what I wanted to want or know. And that is the exact 'rant' I would repeat over and over again when I first began my foray into spirituality – "I want to know what I want to know". I guess in one way I had the perfect canvas to grow into, a blank one. On the outside anyway, but that's okay, I've got a lifetime to continue to grow and sometimes an old pattern will reveal itself for me to recognise and release.

TWENTY-THREE

SEXUAL HEALING – A JOURNEY

With such disruption and distortion in my sexual creative centre, coupled with the old religious beliefs of growing up in a Catholic household, the weight of society's constant opinions of right and wrong, good and bad, self-shaming and guilt, I wanted to learn how to heal myself and others on a deeper level that involves understanding our sexual energy, and how to utilise and develop it in a more loving and healthy way. I didn't know I wanted to know all of this, but I knew that there had to be more for me to learn and to incorporate in my own journey and that of my clients. With this in my psyche, the seed of desire planted, it wasn't long before I knew exactly where I wanted to go. As always, the doors opened up around me and the pull was very strong to learn the art of giving and receiving, next level.

It was a Tuesday evening and there was a new woman who had been invited by one of my clients. I like to welcome everyone and ask them if they would like to share a little about themselves to us. She told the group that her passion was giving a particular style of Hawaiian massage and went on to explain a little about it. We learned that 'Ka Huna' massage is a beautiful and rhythmic massage known to have a deeply relaxing and healing effect. It is at the heart of an ancient healing system developed by the native Hawaiians. 'Ka Huna' and 'Lomi Lomi' massage were used traditionally for ritualised Rites of Passage. For example, it might be performed on the day before a couple was to be married to provide deep healing and open the heart and body to receive the blessings of entering their life together.

I first heard of this technique from a client of mine who was a practitioner. Without even receiving a massage from her, I knew immediately that I had to learn this technique and offer it to clients.

So, in 2016 I flew to the hinterland of Noosa on the Sunshine Coast of Queensland Australia to complete my initial training. Seven days filled with rituals, dances, learning techniques, giving and receiving massage, learning the principles, values and deep spiritual values behind the technique and knowing what a revered and sacred ritual it is to give and to receive.

Our days began at 5am with an optional sauna/cold plunge ritual for half an hour, followed by exercise on the grounds overlooking the beautiful valley below, often with a morning mist lingering above the grass, resembling a mysterious otherworldly presence announcing the rising of the sun. The day was filled with learning techniques in morning and afternoon sessions, meditations to dive deep into spiritual work to help us all access a deeper level of ourselves, homemade vegetarian food to nourish our bodies, time to connect with others in group activities designed to enlighten and enrich our experience, and finally lights out by 10pm. I was lucky to last that long.

During that week I learned so much about giving and receiving in such an intimate and loving way. This massage technique is like no other I have experienced. It can be very sensual since the strokes are long and rhythmic, unlike the usual remedial massage to relieve knots of muscle tension, and often quite painful and intense. It is actually designed to awaken the senses, taking the receiver beyond the busy mind and into their inner world. It is a touch that is so often missing from everyday life, and we can become desensitised through not receiving such intimate loving touch, even though we crave it, since it is easy to resort to quick fix practices to satiate our deep desire for touch.

It was actually quite confronting and a little uncomfortable for me to receive at first. My body wanted to tense, and I felt naked, not only in my body but in my vulnerability. I thought I was here to learn something magical to bring my clients, but it was to learn so much more about myself too. I was drawn to examine where I had been taking shortcuts and accepting less than what I longed for, to satisfy my inner most desires, something so deeply embedded through the busyness of life, coupled with the fear of what is actually lurking deep in my soul that might cause disruption in my ordered life, the life that I had built that was safe and secure.

During the course we were speaking about the reality of the nature of the technique, in that it quite often leads to sexual arousal, and some students were quite disgusted, outspoken and openly put off by this. It's funny how so many women immediately respond with disgust when confronted with the instinctual sexual response, reaction and desire of men outside of the safety of the bedroom. Arousal is a natural response when being touched so sensually, but it 'raised' the question of what to do when that happens.

We were instructed, in alignment with the values of the practice, to be very clear that it wasn't a 'happy ending' massage and to work around any erections that got in the way, using our own discretion when choosing what to say. Since there is only a small modesty towel, and often no towel at all used in this technique – depending on the preference of both the practitioner and the client – it is a technique in which the practitioner must be absolutely clear with boundaries when it comes to options for the receiver. There is a fine line between having a heavenly experience and feeling ashamed for being human and responding from a completely exposed state.

For me, this was going to be quite confronting. My whole language around sex was distorted. I had experienced so much pleasure from sex over the years and really grown from the heightened places it took me, and I had also taken sex and used it to hide from my deepest pain and fears. One minute I could view sex as the most incredible gift we could have been given, and another I could be feeling shame and withdrawal in my body, closing off to being able to view it as anything other than dirty or abusive and disgusting.

It reminds me of a scene in the movie *Something's Gotta Give*. Diane Keaton's character is in love with Keanu Reeves' character, who is much younger than her. She comes to him after finishing a screenplay she had been working on, and they celebrate, he is so proud and in awe of her genius, he pulls her to him, she responds with passion, pulls away, comes in again, pulls away – she is so torn, feeling completely desired but not quite believing it is happening so backs away from him, and, running playfully after her (she is laughing). He says, "Does it always have to be like this?" and I get that, like one hundred percent I get that. It's like there is the most sexual, sensual, sacred feminine residing within me, and her nemesis is the guilt and shame ridden victim who cannot possibly feel desired from her place of deep unworthiness and dishonour.

It is only when I outline my own sexual experiences that I can begin to uncover and possibly understand why this is so, and then delve into the journey of undoing the laces and strings, breaking through the webs, cutting the cords, unlocking the bolted rusty padlocks, and calling out the lies and stories for what they are – deception and fear. While I have had countless and mostly incredible and beautiful experiences, I don't want to underestimate the love and desire and euphoria I have shared, I have also experienced naïveté, been a willing victim to unwanted advances, endured acts where I was gagging, hurting, extremely uncomfortable, humiliated, and downright raped while in a relationship.

I couldn't ignore any longer the calling to not only understand the depths of sexual energy and power, but to heal through utilising sexual empowerment and understanding. And to heal not only myself but as many others as I could through this higher understanding and learning – knowing there is always a higher level of wisdom to attain, since our desire and pleasure knows no limits.

Upon completion of the course, I headed straight to the Gold Coast where I was spending the next four hours with a tantric priestess, learning the art of tantric massage. I had booked this session with her well in advance since I was going to be in fairly close proximity. I had flown interstate to do my KaHuna certification, so it made sense, and I preferred to learn in person rather than online. I had no idea then how perfect it would be.

I arrived at her apartment where we got to know each other in person, having only spoken via messages previously. After about 30 minutes, our volunteer male arrived, I'll refer to him as Mr X, even though I'm sure he would be very open to be identified because he is such an advocate for this work, and continues to work coaching men to become more expanded versions of themselves through movement and sexual understanding on this deeper spiritual level. We eased our way into becoming familiar enough to be vulnerable for the session that would follow. We didn't rush this time of connection, it was imperative to lead into a space of trust, respect and support.

It reminds me of the ancient practices and rituals that I have since looked into. The giving and receiving of sexual pleasure outside of marriage, by highly trained, skillful consummate professionals was not only tolerated and accepted, it was regarded as crucial, indeed the very basis of gaining enlightenment and a deeper connection with the Divine Feminine within. Young women were trained from a very young age with the privilege of bringing this practice to men, just as young men were also shown the techniques to bring a woman into a place of divine receptivity and connection with the Divine masculine within. Sex was sacred. Women would arrange for their husbands to visit these highly respected women when they recognised their husband was needing direction or experiencing stress, worry or anxiety. It was for the benefit of not only their livelihood, but also for their marriage.

The Japanese still openly practice the honoured tradition of the Geisha, a wonderful example of carrying no shame around this practice.

When the time was right, we prepared organic coconut oil by warming it, and went over the tools that are helpful when giving this massage – lubricant, feathers, silk scarves, scented candles or oils, soft music, a comfortable temperature, tissues and towels. I watched my teacher work through the stages, step by step, of breaking down any barriers of fear and expectation, creating a comfortable position for the two of them to sit facing each other, with me sitting close as well, they were supported by cushions on a large bed, fully clothed.

There was a beautiful flow which began with eye gazing, then holding hands, incorporating breathing techniques, silence, deep expression, more silence. I learned where to place my hands to connect the heart and the sexual expression/creative centre, how to encourage the flow of energy to open up the portals that have held blockages. I learned just how much love can be opened up by simply holding space, listening, breathing, gazing and removing expectations. I was beginning to see so much beauty in what was happening in front of me, that in the past I would have been rushing with foreplay, therefore bypassing the most intensely beautiful aspect of connection I was witnessing. I thought I knew how to please men, and I was learning that I knew very little when it came to accessing the sexual pleasure centre through the heart in its most vulnerable and open state.

My preconceived beliefs were debunked, as were the myriad of times I thought that once orgasm was achieved that was the holy grail. How many times had I focused just on orgasm and not on the magic all around it. I was learning how to access a deeper experience of euphoric pleasure via the heart. I was learning that without the heart, in this expanded state, the entire experience is 'less than'. Once you begin to experience vulnerability on a level of complete trust and openness, you let go of inhibitions, bottled up tension and expectations, and then the most wonderful thing happens, you go into the emotions behind the protective walls of your heart.

I learned that holding space is a thing. It's probably the most important thing we can all do in all of the relationships we have, and more so with our intimate partners. As I watched first, and then changed places with my coach so that I was working directly with Mr X, I found myself becoming more understanding of the masculine energy, and it began a process of wanting to dive more deeply with my own experiences, as well as learn as much about men as possible. I wanted to hear their pain, their stories, everything that they felt they couldn't share for fear of being seen as a pussy, (I'll never understand why this word is used in such a derogatory way to display weakness in men) I wanted to hold them while they felt safe to cry or just be still.

As the session progressed, Mr X moved to the massage table and lay on his stomach, and following the guidance of my coach, I used some of my newly learned massage techniques, incorporating the soft touch of feathers and silk, light fingertips and soft blows through my lips all over his body, learning the most sensual areas as I kept the channel of communication open by asking every now and then how he was feeling, and to let me know if he didn't like something I was doing.

After a while I asked him to turn over and I began the same process on the front of his body. At this stage I was interested to see that he didn't have an erection, since with a regular foreplay massage it would normally be all about arousing him sexually. He was quiet and reflective and enjoying feeling the sensations all over his body, so the energy wasn't directed only to his sexual centre. He was feeling pleasure everywhere, as well as going into some deeper emotions that became heightened through loving touch and an atmosphere of support and love.

What I was learning and what he was experiencing wasn't about an end result, not at all, not even a little bit. It was of no consequence whether he had one or more orgasms, or none at all. I was learning that a sexually awakened man, a man who explored his body and sexuality with curiosity such as he did, had no destination when it came to intimacy. Ejaculation was not a priority or even on the radar, as he explored the deeper layers of his mind body spirit connection.

I learned the art of lingam massage. I had never explored a man's penis in this way before, nor viewed it as the 'wand of light', as described in tantric terminology. It was as if, through the sacred and respectful process we were honouring, that my whole views were changing, for the better. I could feel so much restriction, judgment and expectation lifting from my mind. This was magical. In giving this pleasure, I felt incredibly honoured and so trusted. I had never thought of exploring so many varied ways of stroking and playing like this, so much variety when you learn how to approach the frenulum, the foreskin if there is one, the head of the penis, every aspect and angle loves being touched.

And it was about to go a step further, something that I had never explored before, something that I always viewed as out of bounds, dirty and if I'm being honest, disgusting. I was going to explore his greatest area of receiving pleasure, his prostate. We took so much time, care and constant checking in as we went through this process, it felt like a privilege for me to learn that there was no shame to be held around the anus and prostate, although this has continued to be an ongoing learning experience for me since I've only really ever heard the very negative aspects of anal sex.

The prostate is the male g-spot, and men are missing out on another world of pleasure when they and/or their partners hold such shameful emotions around this area. I found the prostate quite easily given the amazing guidance from my coach, and explored tenderly with constant checking in with Mr X. There are many variations in exploring the prostate and it can be incorporated with stroking the penis or testicles as well.

A crucial aspect around this exploration and education was to learn that the prostate is where tons of emotional baggage is stored. Anger, grief, betrayal, guilt and shame can all be hidden, so when it is stimulated in this way, and in an environment that is conducive to feeling safe, a tidal wave of emotions can erupt. Therefore, as a sexual experience, it may well be the gateway to healing and even moving to another level not only in the relationship with a partner, but with self. There are sex toys designed specifically for men to be able to access the prostate since it's pretty challenging to connect with it if you're inflexible, overweight or not quite sure what you're looking for.

I had experienced a life changing and life enhancing week, and it was pretty overwhelming. When I planned the trip, I didn't realise the significance in joining the two modalities I had just learned and how I would dearly want to educate men and women alike on pleasure as a form of healing and growing. It certainly made me look very deeply at my own discombobulated beliefs and stories.

I had a deep desire to work with men, in creating a safe and healing space where they could receive healing, massage and optional tantric massage. I thought I would be adding to the current healing and transformational sessions I already did. However, I now know that it's not what I feel comfortable or called to offer as a service, I prefer to keep this sacred practice for my own intimate relationships, and honestly, it has completely changed the way I am in a relationship. Not to mention how it is received! Not many men have been touched in this way before, nor have they experienced sacred sex from a heart connection, from a woman who is totally present and void of expectations, and instead listening and moving around his body with awe and a confidence that is sensual and very sexy.

I'm now so passionate that I'll talk about this to anyone who desires to know more and provide specific sessions around the practice. I have worked with couples who have incorporated these practices into their relationship with incredible results. The initial and most epic results happen not from the specific sexual practices, which definitely happens but can often happen over time, but rather when communication is addressed in a way it hasn't been addressed before, that's when the magic begins.

Despite my reluctance to expose myself in extolling the virtues of things such as prostate and lingam (penis) massage, I was told by my mentor that I was to just do it. She instructed me to make a video for my Facebook group on the precise subject of prostate massage. I tried to worm out of it and ended up doing a very watered-down version. When I reported back to her, she lost it! The task was specific, and I chose to ignore the very advice I was paying her for. That's what old beliefs and fears will do, steer you away from the very things that raise fear and judgment, the actions that you know will raise eyebrows or have people talking about you behind your back.

I learned that you can do all the courses in the world, work with the best coaches and trainers, read every book that has all the answers you need to go next level with your life, but you can always choose to play down the message, reason with yourself and your supposed limitations, and get lost in the old patterns and self-talk that keep you stuck, reading the next book, doing the next course. I was done with playing small and decided to act on her instructions, precisely, not half arsed.

So, I set the scene and made some mental notes, and ad-libbed my way through a descriptive video on Facebook, and then shared it to YouTube. Well it began receiving some attention, then more attention, and then I began seeing my subscriber list grow into the hundreds, and each month the views were increasing. Wow, I couldn't have dreamed that I could raise so much awareness in men. Of course, there have been some crude comments, some marriage proposals, but the majority of comments have been so positive and encouraging it's been overwhelming. As I write this one year after posting the video, it's sitting at over 100,000 views.

The thing is though, I got stuck. How could I possibly follow up with something as epic as this? I have remained stuck but am now taking action to go to the next step and swallow down the fear of being a fraud and a one hit wonder. It's time to add my next video regardless of the outcome. I don't want to be like Harper Lee, the author of *To Kill A Mockingbird* which was published in 1960. The success of this masterpiece kept her from publishing more work, surely, she thought, she would be judged for each forthcoming piece of work, always being compared to her debut Pulitzer Prize winning novel. Her second novel was finally published in 2015 – fifty-five years later – and one year before her death, and it was actually written before her first book.

Harper Lee is a larger than life example, but it works for me, and if you can use it to propel you to your next masterpiece, whatever that may be, I hope it's helpful! One year is enough to procrastinate, and by the time this book is published I know I will have gotten out of my own way enough to let my next projects come to life, without judgment or expectation, those silent thieves of creativity.

TWENTY-FOUR

DATING IN THE MODERN WORLD

There is so much judgment around online dating, and I was one of the biggest snobs around it. To me, it was absolutely okay for anyone else to do it, but I would never go there, I had a brick wall around other people knowing I needed to look online for a date. It seemed humiliating and embarrassing and like I had failed in some way to actually resort to going online. Well, in January 2016, four years after my fifteen-year relationship and marriage had ended, I created an account and very quickly met a few men. With my history of falling very quickly for a man and being blinded by infatuation, it certainly didn't fail to provide me with some stories to tell.

I had no idea of the games played online as far as dating is concerned. So many men, and women for that matter but I'm focusing on men here, aren't being truthful in the least of their intentions. I've found that a large percentage of men are recovering from divorce/separation from long term relationships and have had their confidence ripped from them. They haven't done any sort of emotional or healing work on themselves and then go online into a world of brutal exposure and rejection. I get this, because options for a healing process after divorce are practically nonexistent and definitely not spoken about much at all. It's usually something like, "Now that I'm free from that, I'm fine and ready to move on."

This thinking is so out of alignment with what needs to be done on a heart and soul level, that it's akin to having third degree burns and then just splashing water on them. The wounds go deep from any major relationship breakdown, and I've found that the shallowness I saw in men was attributed to a deeper fear of being emasculated, abandoned, not being seen or appreciated, and feeling used. Many men I went on dates with had come out of almost sexless relationships, sometimes having to beg for sex, but the one resounding element that was missing in 100% of those men, was intimacy – not sex, intimacy, the difference is monumental. Men crave intimacy every bit as much, and often more than, women.

During these past years I have continually been working on myself with regard to healing, learning and growing from immersing myself in deep cleansing meditations, visiting places where I've been called in order to attain a deeper understanding of my soul journey here, choosing to cut ties with certain people and old stories and beliefs I've been carrying around for way too long.

I recognise that this is something not a lot of people consciously set out to do, so my own expectations when it comes to others have been sorely unfulfilled. I've dated men from all walks of life – an engineer, a lawyer, a professor and author, a tennis coach, a high end restaurant manager, two self-made millionaires, an executive in between jobs, a photographer, a real estate agent, an airline pilot, a salesman; they have ranged in age from 25 to 55 years old and in nationality from Australian to British, African American, French, South African and Italian. They have all been very attracted to finding out more about me and have mostly been intrigued by the work I do and have done on a personal level, but they haven't been very open to actually exploring deeper spiritual work on themselves.

Sometimes they would say that what I do is exactly what they need, and almost make a commitment to themselves that they will begin that inner journey, but it hasn't ever lasted. I get that, it's intrusive and a vulnerable path to open up to, and the armour we build around ourselves is often solid.

It's a brave and timely decision to walk the path of opening up to that kind of vulnerability, but I guess that coming from the perspective where I have been and recognising it in them too, I see the pain behind the walls. In fact, I don't want to work with someone in that way if I'm in a romantic relationship with them anyway, it's not a good way to begin a relationship, in my opinion.

Old habits are hard to break, and that continued proving itself time and again because I found myself stepping away from my own opinions many times, in order to validate theirs. I am not available for that anymore, and this is the biggest lesson I have learned from the whole experience so far – the fine art of recognising true care and compassion from the subtle art of people pleasing that's so easy to fall into.

With feminism so prevalent, it's very important to me to know when I'm getting close to saying something that will emasculate a man, because I believe they have received way too much of that in a manner that many women don't realise they are doing it. The small things that make a man feel desired, needed and loved can often be very quickly turned around with a remark that deflates him, leaving him in a place of not even wanting to try anymore. It's subtle and women often wonder why he switches off so quickly after a little jab, but it goes deeper than surface level. Alison Armstrong has been one of my greatest teachers in this field, having started learning though her first book *The Queen's Code*, I highly recommend it for men and women alike.

The pattern that I fell into when I got back into dating was being available for a man whenever he chose. I would literally drop things, change appointments, rearrange my schedule and anything else I could do, to make myself available for when they wanted to see me. I hadn't really come very far at all in this area, sadly. So, I ended up attracting men who were wanting a Clayton's relationship, yes, remember the advertising for Clayton's? The drink you have when you're not having a drink, right! So, like a drink with no alcohol in it, I was entering into relationships with no responsibility.

I found myself having private trysts and rendezvous and enjoying often amazing sex, but not an outing or dinner invitation in sight. Still, I made excuses and waited for him/them to be ready to go next level, always making excuses to my friends and family that he was so busy and travelling and all the things, when actually, he was getting exactly what he wanted, satisfaction and intimacy, with zero commitment, and no, his family didn't even know about me. I wasn't looking for a ring or marriage proposal, but I was looking for a partner to share my life with on a larger scale than the confines of the bedroom. The issue here? As has been my pattern time and again, communication, AND learning the language that men speak is entirely different from the language women speak.

Women tend to believe that men say one thing but actually mean something else. For example, he might say that he doesn't have room in his life right now for a relationship because work is his top priority. A woman will very likely turn this into a plethora of possibilities that he is not saying, like: he's saying that but he's really just leaving the possibility open, so I'll work harder to prove that I'm perfect for him and then he will realise he does have time for a relationship. No. He is actually saying what he means because he has thought about it and this is the actual decision he has come to. It doesn't matter how much you want him to commit to you, work less, change his mind, he is being honest with you and expects that you will respect that. We expect men to behave like women behave in so many circumstances, but like Alison Armstrong says, men aren't just hairy women, they have an entirely different program running than women do.

I'm not down on myself for taking so much time to learn the importance of communication from my place of not wanting to upset the status quo, or to appear needy, controlling or emasculating. For me, that's what this life is all about, learning, then integrating as much as you can, or at least as much as you're ready for, into your life. I believe I've been doing this, and I have and continue to experience more and more fulfilling relationships on all levels because of it, not least of all with my family. Improved relationships can look like spending more time apart from someone, not talking as much and therefore benefitting more from less. I'm also a great believer that we are here to teach what we are here to learn, so it makes perfect sense to be taking baby steps myself, while being able to watch others around me, including many, many clients, take their relationships next level with the art of communication.

My clients have different attachments to old stories, beliefs and patterns than I do, and they will progress at the pace they are ready for, letting go of all that baggage either instantaneously or progressively, but always seeing enormous shifts. Being used to a certain behaviour and getting attention in a certain way from others can be a catalyst to not even wanting to let go and move on to a happier place. Each of us is responsible for our own pace, it's not on anyone else, so that means we cannot place blame on a person or situation that we're unwilling to either acknowledge or shift.

With my particular skills or gifts, I can tap into the field around others and see the gaps, the messy knots, and the mismatched codes in their field. I love starting the process of unravelling and reconnecting the codes, mostly because of the stories that come back of the unexpected changes they experience, there is a sequence to this process and it's different for everyone.

Acknowledging a communication disruption is only the beginning though, since it will open up a multitude of pathways to explore when it does open up. We can often make the mistake of talking things through, but not know how to go beyond the point where things become stuck again. Changes may happen, but old habits return. I've definitely been there, and I have had sessions with marriage counsellors, none of which I have had good experiences with. For me, I have seen firsthand the enormous gap in what counsellors are taught to help people, and what actually helps, and that's because it's not in their books.

Clinical psychology only touches the surface. My opinion is that it must be blended with other methods of healing to have any lasting or positive results. We can all learn methods to do any number of things, but it's up to us to implement them, and that's where the traditional "counselling by the book" falls short. Most people are unable to embody the changes required because the roots run so deep, they will carry old patterns through to future relationships, jobs and financial situations.

Conversely, counselling may be extremely helpful to shift something that's in the way before you can get deeper into the real healing work. It's all about the layers, and how willing we are to shed them.

There is a paradigm shift happening, and in these years of instant gratification we are seeing so much spirituality thrown around. From the meditation retreats, to walking on fire ceremonies, the five steps to this and ten steps to that, the journaling and the social media darlings with the millions of followers who hang off their every word and mimic their lifestyle choices when it suits them. This silent roar shows the deep yearning that everyone has for meaning and for direction and to make sense of a longing inside to discover more to life.

My advice, through my own experience, is to feel into what is helpful to you in the now, but don't cling to it as the thing that will always be right for you because it's about growth, not stagnating in a safe place.

Is life fair?

Do we attract everything we experience, even the bad stuff?

I look at it this way. If everything is energy, which it is, then if we close off our senses to only allow ourselves to FEEL what is around us, we would surely lead an entirely different life. Our senses highlight the energies with embellishments to make them appear different from what they really are. Like looking at an image in a picture and seeing the absolute beauty in it, and then seeing it in an expanded version and it's not at all what you thought. Like seeing a person on social media living the perfect life that you dream of, even envy and finding out how unhappy they really are. We are surrounded by illusions and they protect us most of the time, which is good, but when is it time to lift the veil, to unlock the vault of half-truths and reveal them fully? That's up to you, to all of us.

TWENTY-FIVE

BREAST IMPLANTS – WORST DECISION EVER

"You are perfect, just as you are."

For years I had joked with my friends and kids that one day I'd get implants. Then in November 2011, just months after my marriage had ended, I had an unexpected windfall, and in that moment, I decided I would look into having implants. Everything happened like a whirlwind after that, and I was excited to feel voluptuous and really sexy. It was like a reward for having breastfed four babies for a year each, I thought my breasts would look fuller and I could say goodbye to padded bras. I went with a recommendation from a friend from the gym who had just had her surgery and seemed really happy with the result. So, I called and arranged for my initial consultation with this popular plastic surgeon.

The appointment went seamlessly, and when asked to choose the cup size I wanted to have, the nurse and the doctor both swayed me to go for the larger size than I originally asked for. I wanted a B cup – nothing too outrageous or different than my current frame, but they convinced me to go for a large C cup. It turned out that I would be wearing D cup bras, something I didn't want but I believed them when they told me that everyone who goes small always wishes they went larger. In fact, it was like playing a game when I went for my pre surgery appointments, all excitement and smiles and laughs. I never once entered into a conversation with any of the staff or the surgeon about the potential risks (other than the surgery itself) or any possible adverse after-effects. I didn't do my own research either, which was definitely a massive oversight.

Surgery was on 22nd December 2011. My daughter dropped me off and went to work, where she waited for the call to come and pick me up. There was an issue with me waking up from the general anaesthetic, and when I eventually remember coming to, I felt like I just wanted to sleep forever, I resisted waking up but I knew I had to. My poor daughter was worried sick and so relieved when she finally got the call, many hours after the scheduled time.

My recovery was going well over the following week, I was taking it super easy, as instructed. Then on day eight post surgery, I was sitting on the toilet and felt a sensation in my right breast, then began feeling off. I got up and headed straight for the bed because I felt like I was going to faint. I grabbed my phone from the bedside table, thinking I might need it close to me if I didn't feel better shortly. The pain got worse and I noticed my breast on that side began swelling slowly, it became too painful to move even slightly. Even though we were separated I called my husband, and he came straight away, hearing it in my voice that I was far from okay.

He called the nurse, who asked him to send through photos. Indeed, it was swelling even more, eventually to around twice the size and the pain was excruciating, so I contacted the surgeon. He had already left for his holidays up the coast, a few hours' drive away. He instructed her to ask me to admit myself to hospital the next morning when he would drive back to drain the area of fluid. This wasn't good enough, and since I was in so much pain, we drove to the hospital where I admitted myself that afternoon and was hooked up to a pain killer via an intravenous drip until the surgery the following morning, New Year's Eve.

The surgery went well apparently, he drained 500ml of fluid from the area, having to completely remove and replace the implant. Thank goodness, the relief was so good when I woke up, and I didn't have the issue with the anaesthetic this time.

As I continued with my recovery, with the loving care of my daughter Angela who nursed me during the following week – I'm not sure just how I would have fully recovered so well if it wasn't for her doing everything for me so I didn't have to lift a finger – I got pretty down on myself. What was I thinking, having unnecessary surgery, and why was I not satisfied with my body? I wished I hadn't done it, I was remorseful and felt ashamed that I had been so selfish to my family, putting them through this. The regret was real, also because my breasts were now looking so large, compared to the itty-bitty ones I had always had.

This time I healed fully, and a few months later I was training again, but didn't feel that I could resume lifting weights until many months later. I got used to the new me in the breast department and began even liking them a bit more.

The downside, other than the initial regret, was that I had no feeling at all in my nipples, and this was pretty devastating for me, I had always been so sensitive in that area, it played a large part in my sex life. The feeling returned after a couple of years, though still not fully. In hindsight, I would have looked much more carefully into all of the changes that I would experience.

Life went on, and I focused on my health especially since I had been anaemic for a few years, so I focused on turning that around even though I didn't really see big results in my energy levels. I did a lot of work on myself and my spiritual world opened up, my life was looking great.

As the next few years went by, I noticed sharp pains in my breasts, intermittently, but definitely not very comfortable at all, not so painful as to require painkillers or to even mention it, but more like recurring short bursts of pain as the time went on. My energy levels should have been getting better since my iron levels were beginning to improve and were better than they had been for many years. Still I felt fatigued, and my eyesight continued to deteriorate with each optometrist visit.

In hindsight, which is the only thing I can rely on now, I began to accept the low energy as a permanent thing, always blaming it on my iron levels being low again, however I was sick of getting blood tests all the time, robbing me of my precious iron so I just got on with life. And getting on with life with low energy meant learning to live with much less life force than I knew I had. I had given up the sport of triathlon very soon after my anaemia diagnosis in August 2005, simply because I became so tired, I couldn't train at all.

It was then that I took up the bikini competition training for two years, and even though I trained well, I needed so much recovery time and it drained me for the normal things in life as well. By this stage I was very good at faking my energy levels because I was sick of being so tired and drained all the time. I just sucked it up and tried to convince myself that I had more energy than I did.

The next few years saw me complete my personal training certification and begin taking clients on health and wellness journeys, focusing on losing weight and gaining healthy lean muscle mass. I loved it, however brain fog kept on settling in during my sessions with clients, particularly in late afternoon or early evening sessions. My eyesight was getting worse and I was so tired all the time. I recall many sessions where I was barely able to comprehend what the client was saying, and I had to blink often to stop myself staring into space. It was awful. I didn't want to be there because I was so very exhausted, yet I loved the work I was doing, it was a conundrum.

I didn't link any of this fatigue and brain fog and blurry vision to my implants, I actually put it all down to my low iron levels which results in almost identical symptoms. But according to detailed blood analysis two years ago my iron levels elevated and returned to a range on the low end of normal, even so, I still believed it would somehow be related to iron levels.

Then one day one of my daughter's friends began posting on social media about breast implant illness (BII) awareness. I looked into her posts and initially thought she was overreacting, surely it wasn't a thing. My reaction says so much about the lack of information available regarding the negative and deadly effects of breast implants.

A few months went by, and she had her surgery to explant her implants, which I didn't even know was a thing, let alone there was a name for the surgery. I talked to her when we were at my daughter's hens party and she elaborated on some of the alarming effects of breast implants. She was due for surgery in the coming weeks and was visibly upset, going through so much emotional turmoil around the whole journey she was still on. She told me she regretted having her implants when she was only 19. She told me that now that she had three young boys and a husband, she wanted to be around for a very long time and wasn't about to risk having ticking time bombs in her chest.

She had found out about the cancer BIA ALCL – Breast Implant Associated Anaplastic Large Cell Lymphoma – that can form particularly from textured implants. It has claimed lives in many countries, yet the offending implants have only been banned in very few countries because the awareness isn't there. She was terrified about developing cancer and having no symptoms until it was too late, hence her decision to have the explant surgery.

I have found even saline implants aren't safe. Most surgeons will tell you they are completely safe, as my surgeon did, and even if they rupture the fluid will be readily absorbed by the body. The thing they omit from that conversation is that the outside of the implant is silicone, and often textured and this will naturally flake and leach out and into the 'capsule' (the protective layers of skin that grow around the implant) and possibly migrate further into your lymph system over time. The capsule is where most of the dangerous toxins lie, but they are not always retained just there. The leakage of toxic metals and poisonous substances somehow find their way around the body often resulting in symptoms that mimic autoimmune diseases, yet no traditional markers appear in blood tests hence why many women are told it's psychosomatic, all in their head, and you guessed it, usually by male surgeons.

My initial appointment with my augmentation surgeon in Double Bay was on December 16, 2019. My daughter accompanied me, which is so poignant since she is the one who nursed me in the beginning, and has supported me in every decision I've made, especially on this journey of discovery. This surgeon's professionalism is second to none, and that is why I chose to return to him, at least for this informative appointment. All of my initial surgery details including before and after photos had been previously emailed to me upon request and we were now looking at them in his rooms. I had some more photos taken before he came in to see me. Since he knew my intention to explant, he welcomed any and all concerns and questions I had.

Why was I choosing to explant? He wanted to know my concerns and reasons. I told him about the awareness I had recently been drawn to and the numerous cases I had seen of the devastating effects of BII. I told him of the symptoms I believed may be attributable to BII and he listened. He explained that the autoimmune type of symptoms that appear in women with BII mostly resulted in no markers in the pathology, however the society of plastic surgeons as a whole have agreed and accepted the belief that, despite scientific proof, the symptoms were real, and the care of these patients was top priority.

However, when I raised the concern that the outer lining of the implant contained silicone, he laughed and dismissed it as false, making me feel a bit silly. My concurrent research has found out that he is the one that should feel stupid, laughing at me when I was speaking the truth. Why doesn't he know these things?

Then he dropped a bombshell.

My implants have been recalled. They are not being used anymore, and removal is recommended. Holy shit! My daughter was horrified and asked why I hadn't been contacted about this immediately. He responded, again with a wry little smile, that unlike a recall for a motor vehicle – yes, his words – there was no obligation to inform patients who actually have the implants, they are just now restricted from being used and have had a recall put in place by the TGA until further information is available to support them being passed as 'safe' once more. So, they're not safe enough to put in because of all the problems i.e. debilitating illness they have caused, but you don't get a courtesy letter to inform you of this. Great.

He went on to explain that even if I wanted to retain my implants, he would strongly recommend that I have them removed as soon as possible. Nine to nine and a half years is around the median time that irregularities and negative health symptoms begin to appear with these implants, so it appeared I was in the right place at the right time. No surprises there since by this stage in my life I know a synchronicity when I see it, and I act on those synchronicities immediately if I feel a call to action. So now I was being given information that, had I not had my recent insight with BII, I would not have been privy to. I would perhaps have incubated mystery illnesses for another five or even 10 years before thinking I needed a review. Even that is being a little generous as to what I probably really would have done, which is to not have followed up at all.

It's not uncommon for women to have implants up to 20 and 30 years with no follow up with their surgeons, no check ups, no MRIs, no ultrasounds. And if there is no responsibility on the manufacturer, like there is with cars, because vehicular faults can cause injury and death directly relatable to the defects, then these implants are purely and simply ticking time bombs in the chests of women around the world.

My decision was made, I wanted to explant as soon as possible. I still wanted my original surgeon to perform the surgery because he was familiar but decided to get a second opinion from my daughter's friend's surgeon. After the consultation with the second surgeon I decided to go with him because his bedside manner was impeccable. He listened without judgment, and gave his opinion based on his experience with previous clients and with his research. And the bonus was that his quote was 60% less than the other surgeon. I'm pretty sure that my original surgeon wanted to get rid of me because I made him face confronting questions about the whole breast enhancement industry and he was almost defensive as well as being the polar opposite of compassionate. But if that's where his thriving business lies then of course, he doesn't want word spreading about the adverse effects that so many women encounter.

My second appointment was with a highly recommended surgeon who was highly skilled in explant surgery. I had discovered him through a Facebook group providing unbiased information, as well as before and after stories from women experiencing issues, and having explant surgery. My initial appointment confirmed the knowing that I was going to have this procedure asap. My surgery date was booked for February 11, 2020 and it couldn't arrive quickly enough as far as I was concerned. It seemed that my symptoms were becoming more pronounced. I began seeing that the extreme hair loss I had been experiencing that was growing worse, losing handfuls of hair each time I washed and brushed it. I noticed I always had a rash on my stomach and my breasts were often very itchy. I was so ready for this procedure to be done. My emotions had gone from anger to blame to frustration and then to acceptance of my situation. I could be an example to other women and a voice to speak up about the dangers associated with breast implants.

The day finally arrived, and the surgery went well. The surgeon was able to remove the entire capsule along with the implants. The implants were intact, no leakages or perforations but one was discoloured due to an inflammatory response from my body. In the weeks leading up to surgery I had noticed my left breast seemed swollen, it was uncomfortable and very concerning. Since I was already booked in, I didn't look into this any further, choosing instead to mention it to Dr W on the morning of surgery.

As I was being prepped in theatre, my anaesthetist was beginning his job of intubating me for the cannula. He was finding it difficult to get a good vein, probably because I had been lying and waiting in pre-op for about two hours and was cold. He was so rough that I reacted and told him he was hurting me, only for him to ignore me and continue probing to find an appropriate vein which he prodded and jabbed painfully. It was extremely uncomfortable, and my hand began cramping and as I was telling him this, I drifted off into anaesthesia land. I reported him to my surgeon saying I was disgusted with his behaviour and bedside manner. My surgeon later assured me he spoke with him and would be keeping a close eye on his behaviour.

I posted in the Facebook group to be aware of this guy, and why. One lady was anxious because she was booked with him the following week, so when she spoke to the receptionist, she raised concern. She went on to report back to me that she had the most beautiful experience with him. I don't know, maybe I got him on a bad day, or maybe he just needed a wakeup call to work from his heart and recognise that we put so much trust in his work, and his bedside manner.

When I woke up back in my private room, thank goodness for private health insurance! I immediately felt relieved, lighter and had absolute clarity that I had made the right decision. My surgeon sent the capsules and the fluid he had drained from my swollen breast to pathology, and they all returned with no signs of cancer or abnormalities. The thickness of the capsule indicated that my system had indeed been fighting for quite some time against the silicone and the foreign matter in and around the implant. The surgery had been delicate since the capsule was quite stuck to my rib cage and required precision to remove it as completely as possible without puncturing a lung.

I stayed in the hospital for three nights under the care of some awesome and hysterically funny nurses, all either Scottish or Irish so I loved the accents, and then Ryan, who also dropped me off, drove me home and pampered me over the following days. I may have played on it a little, but it was so beautiful to be so lovingly cared for by him and Daniel.

I returned back to teaching Pilates six days later and my strength and range of motion slowly returned. The scars have healed beautifully, and my follow up appointments have all been positive. I love feeling like the old me again, wearing the tops I used to love without having to dress around a large bust, which I must admit I really loved sometimes, but more often than not, I secretly wished I had never had the surgery in the first place.

As the weeks went by, I was definitely feeling less tired and fatigued, I noticed improvements in my skin and definitely in my demeanour, the depression lifted. Life was so good and in the first few weeks I talked to three women specifically about my experience, and happily those women have chosen to not go ahead with breast augmentation. I openly discuss this journey with anyone who is interested. Word of mouth is the most effective form of communication, particularly with women, and I openly use my platform to educate women on all manner of experiences. In fact, the tabooer the topic, the more I will discuss it openly in class in an inquisitive, informative and respectful way.

TWENTY-SIX
DING DING – WAIT – WHAT?

I continued following the stories of several other women in the Facebook group who were anxious about their upcoming surgeries as well as women who were experiencing recovery, the good the bad and the ugly. One day I happened across a post about surgical clips being left in patients and causing terrible problems with their health, but then a word shouted at me from the page: "Essure". This captured my attention because I had these titanium contraceptive devices implanted in 2004. The more I read, the more I learned about the true cause of my debilitating anaemia which surfaced in the months following that procedure.

I had Daniel at 40 and decided I didn't want to have any more children but was struggling to find a suitable contraceptive, since I didn't want to go back on the pill. I didn't open the topic for discussion with my husband other than to inform him of my preference for the Essure. I actually told him I didn't want him to even consider a vasectomy because if something happened to me then I didn't want him to not be able to have more children, whereas I was certain I had birthed all the babies I had chosen to.

During a visit to my gynaecologist to discuss my options he presented me with not many alternatives other than the usual coil, Mirena and tubal ligation. Then he presented me with an option, something new on the market that he praised, while also warning me it wasn't reversible if I changed my mind and wanted another baby. I was totally sold from the way he described it. Very small titanium coils which are inserted into the fallopian tubes. The effectiveness comes from the scar tissue growing around the devices, preventing the eggs dropping. So, I made my appointment for a day procedure and felt absolutely fine with no down time afterwards.

It's relevant to note here that I had never experienced any issues with my menstrual cycle. I had never had heavy bleeding in the 28 years I had been menstruating, I had occasionally experienced mild cramping when ovulating, but mostly my cycle was regular and fairly light. I had been on the pill intermittently for several years but that didn't really affect my experience of my monthly cycle. Therefore, I had a good knowledge of what my cycle was, both on and off the pill.

During the second month after the procedure I began having very heavy periods, and they became heavier and more uncomfortable each month. I asked my gynaecologist at least twice about this, and his response was similar to my implant surgeon which was initially a "pfft" followed by denial and that it absolutely had nothing to do with the procedure with Essure. I believed him when he told me that as women get older, they often bleed more heavily, that their cycle changes, convincing me that it was my body that had changed dramatically because of, well, nothing.

As I mentioned earlier in the book, my triathlon coach picked up on my pale colour and asked me to have my iron levels checked, which led to the diagnosis of the incapacitating and career destroying anaemia. To give an indication of the amount of blood I was losing, when I got out of a chair I would gush blood, the bedsheets were soaked with my blood for days of my period so I was washing them daily, and getting out of bed was a well-orchestrated plan with towels by my bedside to place like a large nappy, ready for the deluge when I stood up and raced for the shower. There were not pads that were thick enough to absorb the blood flow, and even if there were, the large clots that slid out could not be absorbed, they were just solid.

I still trained throughout all of this, carefully planning enough absorbing protection to last me for the session I was doing, but cycling was the worst. I was lucky the cycle shorts are padded because that allowed me to pad them up even further, and I always wore black because when I got off the bike my shorts would be soaked with blood and the pads were heavy and dripping.

Yes, it was awful, it was extremely embarrassing and I remember once when I snapped at my husband for something silly during my period, because I was so tired all the time, I got cranky, he snapped back at me saying how he wished I would clean the toilet seat better when I had my period. That made me so very upset, because if only he knew how bad it was. I didn't let on to anyone how bad it was, so trying to act normal was a structured process. Getting off the toilet would result in a gush, no matter how long I waited before standing up, which went all over the toilet seat and floor, so I was constantly cleaning up after myself, but I must have left a telling smear now and then. I know, gross, but I was just trying to stem the flow so guess I overlooked the odd smear a couple of times. Again, my poor communication didn't help me out here because I just went away and silently cried in frustration and embarrassment and sadly, even shame.

Does that create a picture of the change in my life after Essure? I'm crying writing this because of the memories surfacing, but if I didn't think it was worth sharing and perhaps even raising awareness, I certainly wouldn't be writing about it.

It wasn't until I had been enduring this for around one year that the anaemia hit, which is when my coach picked up on it. I worked with my GP on iron supplements, iron injections which I reacted badly to, and changes in my diet to try to regain my iron levels. We wanted to approach it without hormone interference and as naturally as possible. I did take a drug that stopped my period just as it was beginning, for one month, but it just didn't seem right, so I didn't continue. He was perplexed since I told him about my concerns about the Essure, but that my gynaecologist had assured me they had nothing to do with it.

I won't go into the whole debate about tragic TGA approvals for toxic and cancer causing implants of all manner, suffice to say that surgeons are mostly just as ill-informed as the general public about the devices they are putting into our bodies, with poorly structured testing, if any. The power of influence marketing and the temptation of incentives has sadly overridden an inquisitive mind in many cases, even with our top surgeons.

Fast forward to today when I still have low stores of iron, so I'm unable to do anything requiring endurance like running a long distance or lifting heavy weights without literally being wiped out for hours afterwards. I haven't experienced heavy monthly bleeding for two years since my body began shifting into the next phase of womanhood where she ceases her reproductive cycle. I guess I thought this might mean my iron levels would begin climbing higher, and they have – slightly.

Having now spoken with several women and listened to stories of women with these devices, I know resolutely that the cause of my menorrhagia, which is the medical term for excessive menstrual bleeding, is the Essure. It is quite possibly and highly likely related to my gum issues too.

Now begins the next step of finding a surgeon to remove them without having a full hysterectomy. The initial steps involve testing to ensure they haven't migrated out of the tubes and into the uterus, or anywhere else in my body which has happened to many women. They have been known to have migrated all over the body, even to the lungs so I'm not risking having another set of time bombs floating around my body. The vast majority of symptoms across the board include iron deficiency and anaemia, blood clots, onset of excessive bleeding, cysts and tumours often spreading all over the entire reproductive system and bowel, metallic taste, PCOS, dental issues, liver problems, vision problems, autoimmune disorders, Vitamin B-12 and D deficiencies, stroke symptoms and on and on and on.

So now to explore the relationship between being a victim of circumstance and choice, and where it fits into my soul's unfolding.

I have written that my body's conditions, specifically anaemia and gum disease and the effect they had on my body, was a sign that I wasn't living in true authenticity and something needed to change in my life in order for me to recover. Then I discovered the true causes of those conditions which were a direct result of having implants surgically placed in my body, leading to leaching of energy in many forms including physical mental and emotional.

It is very easy to become a victim in such circumstances when adverse health conditions appear and point the finger of blame on outside sources, which I have done to an extent, but not to escape the lessons learned due to those conditions. I believe there will always be a source of trigger to awaken us to living in our authenticity if we are not doing so. I had been living mostly in avoidance of communication in difficult situations, in all my significant relationships. I ran away rather than face confrontation in so many circumstances and this resulted in me living under a veneer of guilt, shame and blame which was easily triggered and allowed me to hide in my child, prostitute, victim and saboteur states when I needed to.

The voice of my child would allow me to blame others and say that it wasn't fair that this or that happened to me.

The voice of my prostitute would easily sell myself on some level in exchange for approval, love and inclusion. For example, being agreeable and a yes person even when I knew it didn't feel right, rather than cause an argument or uncomfortable situation to arise.

The voice of my victim would allow me to gain the sympathy and compassion of others, placing me in a false temporary coma of safety and comfort, while avoiding the actual issue which was avoiding tapping into my own truth and convictions, which had become blurry even to me.

The voice of my saboteur allowed me to introduce all the reasons I couldn't speak up, take responsibility, make decisions in fear of looking silly or not trusting more intelligent people or rules, or straying from the way things have always been done.

While I had lived many wonderful years and countless experiences where I had easily accessed the polar opposite of these voices, I had allowed myself to fall into bad habits which were self-destructive. The feelings of failure and lots of guilt and shame that I lived with over secrets I carried with me, was a toxic breeding ground and incubator for the lower vibrational voices to grow in their power. And that power disintegrates life force. The voices of power and authenticity are the voices of the lover, the sovereign, the warrior and the magician.

The voice of my lover knows that I value myself on all levels and will not sell myself short to anyone or anything. My time, my soul, my body are not for sale at any price, not for any reward, not for any temptation.

The voice of my sovereign knows that I decree all that comes into my life and how I respond to it. When life hands me challenging circumstances, I do not bow out by blaming others or hide behind the safety net of not taking responsibility and needing the approval of others or society to make decisions for myself.

The voice of my warrior knows that nothing and no one has power over me, I will not be influenced by others to make choices that go against my authentic self and my truth. I will not be overpowered by the cowering victim of circumstance who blames anything rather than taking action to change my life when needed.

The voice of my magician has the ability to make lemonade out of the lemons of life. Rather than getting lost in excuses and reasoning my magician voice allows me to access my intuition without doubt, and act upon it immediately. Trust is the only option and diving in at the deep end will usually bring me the best outcome, as I have encountered so many times in my life. It's only when I don't trust my intuition by questioning and procrastinate and reasoning until it goes away, that I achieve life's greatest blessings.

It's so easy to logically explain a course of events using tangible reasoning and historical data, but I believe the magic of the unfolding of our lives lies solidly in what we make of the circumstances around us. I have become more congruent with the term 'synchronicity' to describe this since often there is no other reasoning as to how things come to pass.

UNLOCKED

When a door is unlocked, it does not automatically open itself. To become unlocked from your old ways will certainly free you from being trapped in your limiting beliefs and your ingrained behaviours, however it will not take you by the hand and lead you down a path of sunshine and roses. This, you must do yourself.

It requires action to actually take the steps following the unlocking. It takes courage to open the door/s, to walk through them and to bravely face your fears and anxieties that have kept you behind the safely locked doors of your past.

At no time in my life, when I have taken leaps in my growth and development, have I not taken scary, often terrifying action.

Every single time.

In most cases, I have taken the action that had been offered by my intuition for years prior and I had completely ignored, falling back into the safety of my uncomfortable comfort zone. Finally my body took it upon itself to magnify the intensity of my blocked state, through illness and injury.

I have no regrets in life. Quite the opposite. The very fact that I have taken decades to unlock my true gifts and to begin truly living in authenticity in every way, has paved the way for me to continue my work helping others take the shortcuts I ignored.

My kids all have a long-standing joke that I am an expert at taking long-cuts. You see, I love taking back streets to avoid too many sets of traffic lights or heavy traffic or main roads, and often this had taken us on interesting detours that have taken much longer than the short-cut I told them I was taking.

But what I see is that all of them have learned the art of the long cut. It gives you a greater knowledge of your area, the hidden gems that lie in streets you would never have ventured down. We have discovered the most amazing displays of Christmas lights in quiet streets, beautiful hidden parks and parklands, mansions and hidden estates that we never would have known existed, stunning flowers growing wildly, fruit trees we have picked from – all manner of surprises that would have remained untapped to us. All within our own small area of the world.

All too often it's easier to stay on the main roads and remain stuck in the patterns of the world around us, than it is to venture into the wonderland that lies in the uncertainty of taking the short cut with no set directions, except our intuitive compass.

All it takes is the first step.

It's my promise to myself that I listen to my intuition more intently than ever before. But more than that, it's my vow to take the action required to step through the doorway it reveals, releasing the next step, and the next step, and the next step.

It's my intention to always remember that my intuition offers me only one step at a time, and to have the courage to take the action step required, trusting completely in the knowing that it is the directive of my soul.

It's my goal to live my life knowing that there are endless doorways hiding in the shadows behind every challenge and obstacle I will face.

It is my dream that I encourage and guide everyone that I can to live in their integrity, to discover their truth, and to have the courage to create the change in their life needed to do this.

My wish for you, the reader, is that you rise into your greatest life and live in your truest integrity. That you recognise that you hold the power in your hands to unlock and open and walk through any door that you desire.

> You already have the key.
> Your intuition will guide you.
> Trust it.
>
> Carmelle x

ABOUT THE AUTHOR

Carmelle was born in Bulli NSW where she lived until she was 20. She now lives in Sydney with all of her children close by where she enjoys leading an active lifestyle including teaching pilates and barre classes. Passionate about her work and the gift she brings to the world, she lives and breathes this passion every day. Her private sessions are run from her home or online. She has a podcast and YouTube channel where she often posts informative conversations with past clients, and women who have influenced her to be where she is today.

If you have purchased a copy of this book, we would love for you to send us a selfie of you and the book on your preferred platform:

facebook.com/RealDawnBates
instagram.com/realdawnbates
twitter.com/realdawnbates
linkedin.com/in/dawnbates

...so we can thank you in person.

With love and gratitude,
From all at Dawn Publishing

www.ingramcontent.com/pod-product-compliance
Lightning Source LLC
Chambersburg PA
CBHW021022110526
R18276100001B/R182761PG44588CBX00010B/17